QUIT DIGGING
YOUR GRAVE WITH A
KNIFE AND FORK

QUIT DIGGING YOUR GRAVE WITH A KNIFE AND FORK

A 12-STOP PROGRAM TO END BAD HABITS AND BEGIN A HEALTHY LIFESTYLE

MIKE HUCKABEE

GOVERNOR OF ARKANSAS

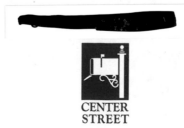

CENTER
STREET

New York Boston Nashville

Center Street
Time Warner Book Group
1271 Avenue of the Americas, New York, NY 10020
Visit our Web site at www.twbookmark.com.

Center Street and the Center Street logo are trademarks of Time Warner Book Group Inc.
Printed in the United States of America
First Edition: May 2005
10 9 8 7 6 5 4 3

Library of Congress Cataloging-in-Publication Data

Huckabee, Mike.
    Quit digging your grave with a knife and fork : a 12-stop program to end bad habits and begin a healthy lifestyle / Mike Huckabee.– 1st ed.
        p. cm.
     ISBN 0-446-57806-1
   1. Weight loss–Psychological aspects.   I. Title.

    RM222.2.H835 2005
    613.2'5–dc22   2004029405

This book is dedicated to my wife, Janet, and my three adult children, John Mark, David, and Sarah, who have seen me at my best and worst and still love and support me; and to the millions of children and adults who, like me, struggle every day with the addiction of eating too much and exercising too little and who have tried to change and cried because they couldn't. It's my hope that within these pages, you will join me in the amazing discovery of regained health by putting a STOP to some bad habits and enjoying the START of healthy living.

You can, and you will!

Acknowledgments

When I'm asked how long it took to write this book, I could say that from the time I wrote the first words until handing over the manuscript to my editors was more than a year, but the honest answer is that it took a lifetime. A lifetime of bad habits and stubbornness brought me to a crisis that would mark the end of "diets" and "programs" and lead to a change of attitude and actions that would save my life. I take full responsibility for sailing into a shipwreck and jeopardizing my very life for the love of food and the loathing of exercise, but the effort to salvage me has many heroes, a few of whom I must acknowledge.

My wife of more than thirty years, Janet, transitioned from chief critic of my bad habits to chief cheerleader for my good ones; my dog, Jet, has been willing to get up with me every morning no matter how early to go for early-morning walks or runs and was actually at my side during the writing of every single word in the text. While he didn't offer much in the form of critique to the concepts or the manuscript, his companionship was invaluable.

My personal physician, Dr. Charles Barg, and his partner, Dr. Torin Gray, were not only my physicians but also my friends as they sat me down for the "talk" to tell me what I had done to myself and what it was going to mean. Their candid but compassionate confrontation was the bucket of cold water that I needed to awaken me from slumber and sloth. Dr. Richard Nix, my orthopedic surgeon, not only coached and counseled me during my early attempts at exercise but also fixed me when I foolishly did too much too soon, and then gave me the green light to take my exercise to a new level–training to run a marathon.

Friends like Arthur (Frenchie) Boutiette introduced me to Dr. Philip Kern of the University of Arkansas for Medical Sciences (UAMS), whose expertise in metabolism and nutrition gave me the initial tools to change. He and his assistant Carolyn Bernthal, RN, a certified nutritionist and dietitian, saw beyond my title of *Governor* and treated me like a patient and client, cutting me no slack yet working with my insane schedule to keep me accountable.

Dawn Cook, my personal assistant, used evenings, weekends, and vacation time to type the early drafts of the manuscript, and her encouragement during the project was as helpful as the typing.

Dr. Fay Boozman, director of the Arkansas Department of Health and a close friend, helped convince me that obesity wasn't only *my* problem, but an epidemic disease that is killing millions of Americans and wrecking the lives of children.

My staff, especially Joe Quinn, policy director, and Chris Pyle, policy adviser for health, shared with me the vision for a "Healthy America," starting with the launch of our state's Healthy Arkansas Initiative.

Dick Dresner, my political consultant, pollster, and personal friend, convinced me to take my experience and share it in book form, and then introduced me to Margret McBride, my agent, who believed in me and believed in "12 STOPS" and, along with a great staff at the McBride agency, pushed it to potential publishers.

Rolf Zettersten, my publisher at Time Warner, has been terrific in shepherding this project from concept to completion and has assembled an absolutely brilliant and genuinely professional team of editors, especially Christina Boys, to make the book much better than I could have.

J. P. Francour, who chairs the Governor's Council on Fitness, has been a godsend, coming over early in the morning on numerous occasions to teach me exercise techniques; his patience is amazing. Geneva Hampton and Gena Marchesse, who operate the Little Rock Marathon, actually talked me into training for the challenging 26.2-mile hilly course, something I would have thought impossible.

The people of Arkansas, my beloved state, have been wonderful and supportive, giving me encouragement at every turn with their kind comments, their affirmation, and the kind of heartfelt support that makes me the most fortunate governor in the nation!

Contents

QUIT DIGGING YOUR GRAVE WITH A KNIFE AND FORK

Introduction

In November 2003, President George W. Bush visited Little Rock for a luncheon speech. As is the case with most presidential visits, his appearance was front-page news the following day. The report included a full-color photograph of the president pointing me out in the crowd and calling me "Skinny."

Having the president of the United States call me "Skinny" in front of a large hometown crowd is nice enough, but having it written in the state's largest newspaper is truly the icing on the cake—even though I don't eat cake anymore!

The president never would have made that statement when he was in Arkansas in November 2002. He had come for the elections and to make a campaign appearance for my reelection bid as governor of Arkansas. That day he certainly *didn't* call me "Skinny," because that was a hundred pounds ago for me.

I can't promise that the front page of your local newspaper will tell your story or that the president of the United States will point you out in a crowded room and call you "Skinny," but I *can* promise that if you faithfully follow the simple, practical, and doable advice you will get in this book, you will be well on your way to what you may have thought would never happen—health and fitness, adding years to your life and a new burst of energy you thought went away somewhere near the time of your senior prom.

If you are one of those people who is looking to lose five or ten pounds before heading off to your class reunion next month, this book won't hurt you. But if your eating habits might well explain the food shortage and hunger problem in third-world countries, this book will teach you how to stop abusing food—and yourself.

I don't ever recall setting a goal to be overweight, but I sure succeeded in getting there!

I went to my doctor, and the diagnosis was fairly simple: "You're fat." Thinking that a bit blunt, I responded, "Maybe I need a second opinion." To which he replied, "Okay, you're ugly, too."

Frankly, I didn't need a doctor telling me that I was approaching the weight of a cement truck. I knew that every time I tried to squeeze into one of the hideously designed aircraft seats in coach or forced myself into a booth in a restaurant where my stomach pressed into the table. Overweight people dread theater seats and especially stadium seats, designed by people with the rear end of a fashion model instead of the rear end of a tractor-trailer rig. Being offered a chair as a guest in a home involves surveying it to determine if it's strong enough to support the weight of two adults, even though only one adult will actually be attempting to sit there.

One of my more embarrassing moments occurred during a meeting of my cabinet in the ornate and historic Governor's

Conference Room on the second floor of the State Capitol. At the appointed time, the door from my office to the conference room was opened by my security detail to signal my arrival. As is custom, the fifty-three cabinet-level agency directors stood as I entered the room and proceeded to the head of the massive table in the center. The conference room had recently undergone a thorough renovation to restore it to its original design. Part of the restoration involved placing antique chairs from the period of the Capitol's construction in the early 1900s around the table.

When I sat in the chair to begin the meeting, I found myself suddenly on the floor. The chair had collapsed underneath my weight. I certainly had everyone's undivided attention! At first there was a collective gasp from those gathered to make sure I was not injured, and then the obligatory comments and concerns were expressed. "Are you okay, Governor? Are you hurt? Would you like another chair?"

I could sense the deep internal tension among those in attendance—somewhere between concern for any injuries and the almost unstoppable instinct to laugh out loud at the sight of the state's chief executive sprawled out on the floor like a scene from a Three Stooges film. I was inclined to cry, realized that it was better form to laugh, and tried to act rather cavalier about the entire episode with a dismissive statement of "Boy, they sure don't build 'em like they used to!"

Deep down, I knew it wasn't the chair that needed rebuilding—it was *me* that needed a major overhaul! Worse than the actual episode was having it captured by security cameras that monitor the room. I am surprised that the tape of that incident hasn't already made its way to *America's Funniest Home Videos* (probably because folks feared that sending it in would make them the newest members of *America's Most Recently Unemployed*!).

It was a humbling—actually a humiliating—moment, and my only consolation was that it happened at a cabinet meeting instead of a press conference with every news organization in the state there to record the sight and sound of the governor destroying a chair and his pride in one single moment!

While that incident was certainly a wake-up call, it was a small part of a larger problem. The fact was, *I was truly sick and tired of being sick and tired*! Maybe you are there as well. You've tried every diet known and still struggle. I have a word for you—STOP! Before you will *start* eating a healthy diet, there are some STOPs to confront.

I haven't always been overweight, but it would be fair to say I've always had a weight problem. Even during those occasional periods in my adult life when I would lose weight, I never made the transition of totally changing my personal habits. As a result, the same bad habits would come creeping back, and with them the same obesity—only usually worse.

In this book, I will discuss why a focus on weight loss will probably lead to failure. Instead, your focus needs to be on actual health and fitness. With permanent health and fitness, the weight will take care of itself, and you will experience liberation from enslavement to what you eat or—better said—to what has been eating you!

I don't have a medical degree, so I won't pretend to offer medical advice. If you want clinical advice given as if in a doctor's illegible handwriting, there are more expensive and much thicker books on the shelves.

While I'm pretty handy in the kitchen and even more so on the outdoor grill, I'm neither a chef nor a nutritionist and will not try to tell you how to prepare wonderful recipes that will make you thin and win blue ribbons at the state fair.

Think of this book as the simple story of *one beggar telling another beggar where to find bread (whole-grain bread, of course!).*

If you are like me, the big issue is not *what* to do but *how* to do it. Even without a medical degree, you already know that reducing calories and increasing physical activity and exercise will result in some degree of weight loss. But while you are aware of this *intellectually*, you have found it difficult to accomplish as a permanent *lifestyle*. That's my story as well.

A Personal Reflection

Like most kids growing up in the South, I was raised to believe that the preferred way of cooking anything is to first batter it in cornmeal or flour and then fry the ever-loving nutrition out of it in a pan of gurgling hot grease. I grew up on fried chicken, fried okra, fried green tomatoes, fried catfish, fried pork chops, chicken-fried steak, fried potatoes, fried onion rings, fried pies, fried squash, and fried ham. Even now, a trip to the state fair will present such "Southern delights" as fried ice cream, fried Oreos, and, yes, even battered and fried Twinkies!

In addition to being Southern, I'm also a Baptist, which means that while we "officially" do not drink alcohol or use tobacco, we are free to eat every kind of food imaginable as long as we fry it and consume it in *large* portions. For those reading this who might live outside the South and cannot fully comprehend what I mean, let me explain from the perspective of a childhood experience. When I was a kid in school, a teacher asked my class to have show-and-tell with the theme being "religion." Children were encouraged to bring a symbol of their faith and explain it to the class. The following day, a Catholic girl brought a crucifix, a little Jewish boy brought a menorah, and I brought a casserole in a covered dish. Get the picture?

In addition to my Southern and Baptist roots, I grew up just a few pocketfuls of change above the poverty level. I had hard-working parents, but their combined income did little more than keep the rent paid and keep food on the table. (Maybe we could have afforded more rent had we not invested so heavily in food.) The food of working-class people is rarely choice cuts of lean meat, fish, and fresh produce. It tends to lean heavily on the kind of dishes that stretch both the dollar and the waistline. Potatoes and gravy are filling and stretch the food dollar. Biscuits and gravy are also cheap and filling. For many poor people, food is the only thing they have in abundance—but only because the really cheap foods can be enjoyed in mass quantities at minimum cost. I was in high school when I realized the reason we ate macaroni and cheese so often was because we were poor, not because we were lucky!

For my entire life, food has been far more than mere fuel for the body. It was what social events were planned around; it was offered to any visitor who came by, even if unexpected or unwelcome. And it was the ultimate medicine for all that ailed.

"You wrecked your bike? Here, have a bowl of ice cream, that will make it feel better!"

That's the way we did things at my house.

"Sit in a bed of ants? Candy bar should fix that, along with a squirt or two of Bactine."

"Did you strike out every time at bat in a Little League game? No problem. We'll stop at the Dairy Queen on the way home and get a chocolate dipped cone." Special occasions were also always marked by a special meal, and not just the obligatory birthday cake once a year. In my family, we *created* events to celebrate with food.

I'm sure by now you're getting the picture. It wasn't hard for me to get heavy. It would have been very difficult for me to be anything else. And let me be both fair and clear—I'm pretty sure that even if my background, upbringing, religion, and culture hadn't contributed to it, I would have ended up that way anyhow, because I just liked to eat! I didn't "eat to live," but I did "live to eat."

Now here's a dirty little secret—many overweight people have a great sense of humor and in fact are often considered "jolly." You know the story—jolly old Santa Claus, his big belly shaking like a bowl full of jelly when he gives out that hearty laugh. But often, fat people are laughing to hide the hurt and humiliation they experience. People constantly make fun of them or, even worse, heap condemnation on them through words, actions, or very obvious attitudes. I found that when I beat people to the punch by making my own jokes about my weight, I was at least able to get the laugh moving on *my* schedule instead of theirs.

So if this has been a lifetime battle for me, what happened to change me? And you may be wondering—how did I lose the weight, and can it work for you?

Yes, if I can do it, anybody can! And—I want you to read this very, very slowly—*so can you!*

In the following pages, I will give you some ideas and some specific instructions on breaking the bad habits and making the new ones as much a part of your life as the old habits were.

Folks who join Alcoholics Anonymous are enrolled in its 12-step program. Twelve-step programs are applied to many addictions, including alcoholism, gambling, sexual activities, drugs, and even smoking.

"Foodaholics" are confronted with a constant craving from their appetite. However, unlike the addictive substances that bring pleasure but are not necessary to sustaining life, food can hardly be sworn off altogether—not if you expect to live.

My experience is that before we can start healthy habits, we have to first break the old ones. And that's the *hardest* part of the battle, and the one this book is all about.

You are about to be introduced to "12 STOPs" toward getting fit. These are specific things that you will need to STOP doing—things that enslave you to a way of life that is destroying your health and self-esteem.

STEPS TO THE STARTING LINE

In 2002, as I was preparing to embark on a long day of speaking and campaigning, I noticed a numbness in my arm and hand that would not go away. At first I thought it was the result of having slept on it during the night. But something just didn't feel right, so I canceled my first event of the day, called my doctor, and described the symptoms. He ordered me immediately to his office. His quick tests revealed what I had dreaded and hoped to have put off for at least another ten or fifteen years: I was diabetic, and my blood sugar was soaring out of control.

I wasn't surprised—I had two parents and two grandparents who were type II diabetic. But I was very angry at myself, because deep down inside I knew this could have been prevented. I knew that this disease diagnosed at the age of forty-seven would probably mean a very strong likelihood of heart attack, stroke, loss of sight, or loss of limb, as well as a much earlier-than-expected death.

I tried to make some adjustments in my life by drastically reducing the amount of sugar I ate and even attempting to cut back on portions. I experimented with several diet plans, most of which involved eating a very specific food or type of food almost exclusively. Nothing seemed to really work, and I hated every minute of it. I felt hungry all the time, deprived and depressed. I was frustrated that while I could succeed in being elected governor and make huge changes in my state, I still couldn't fight off the urge for a doughnut!

During the spring of 2003, while engaged in an especially testy legislative session, I began to experience chest pains and symptoms characteristic of heart disease or blockage in the coronary artery. One night when the symptoms were worse than usual, I called my good friend Dr. Fay Boozman—whom I had appointed director of the Arkansas Department of Heath—and described my condition. He instructed me to go immediately to the emergency room and get checked. I replied that my schedule for the next several days would not allow this and that it would actually be easier to drop dead than to reschedule everything that was on my calendar, but I did promise I would call my doctor and set up an appointment for Friday of that week—four days later. I spent the next four days not only making my way through a long list of scheduled activities, but also contemplating what I was going to find out if I lived long enough to get to the doctor's office by Friday. I did make it to my doctor, who insisted that I go to a cardiologist right away to schedule a heart catheterization. This is a procedure doctors use to view any blockage to the arteries by injecting a dye into the system. Clogged arteries can trigger a debilitating heart attack or even death if not treated.

Prior to having the procedure, I made the mistake of looking at several Internet sites to see what my symptoms would likely reveal. I reached the inescapable conclusion that I did indeed have coronary heart disease and would end up having—at best—angioplasty or—at worst—heart bypass surgery. I was so convinced that I had a heart problem from years of reckless food behavior and lack of exercise that when I went in for my exam, I had already packed a bag that would be appropriate for a several-night stay at the hospital.

Surprisingly, the tests revealed a strong and healthy heart, but the cardiologist pronounced that I was horribly out of shape and told me that without a change of both diet and exercise I would not be able to avoid serious heart and health problems. I was deeply shaken by the experience (which is a nice way of saying I was scared to death!). My primary care doctor, Dr. Charles Barg, sat me down for a heart-to-heart talk and said without major lifestyle changes, I was entering my last decade of life. *I was digging my own grave with a knife and fork!* If I didn't make serious changes in the way I was taking care of my body, I would need to find six very good friends who were fit to be pallbearers for my premature funeral!

Unfortunately, *knowing* we have a problem and even being afraid of it doesn't necessary lead to improved behavior. I had the strongest desire in the world to change, but I thought I had tried everything, to no avail. Sound familiar?

I simply didn't know *how* to succeed.

Not long after this, former Governor Frank White, whom I had appointed state bank commissioner, had announced his retirement and was in my office describing his plans for travel during his retirement years and his anticipation of more leisure time. Less than a week later, Governor White (who had himself become significantly overweight) dropped dead of a heart attack. He was truly one of the greatest people I have ever known. He was a man who found a way to love even those who despised him, and his contagious, larger-than-life sense of humor made him an absolute delight to be around regardless of politics.

It was about this time that one of my close advisers and cabinet members, Arthur (Frenchie) Boutiette, approached me about a weight loss program he was in at the University of Arkansas for Medical Sciences (UAMS) led by Dr. Philip Kern, a renowned endocrinologist whose specialty is research in metabolism. Many people are surprised to learn that UAMS has some world-class medical research programs, especially in geriatrics, oncology, orthopedics, and many others. I was a bit reluctant to try another "diet plan" but also knew that I needed some method to follow, so I decided to inquire about the program. I didn't really expect it to work, either, but *I figured I could die trying or just die dying.* To my relief, and earning my eternal gratitude, Dr. Kern and his nutritionist Carolyn Bernthal took me on. Maybe they needed a challenge!

The balanced and very focused approach of the medically supervised UAMS program has been wonderful, and I have recommended it to many people. The UAMS program approaches weight loss from the perspective of permanent lifestyle change through developing healthy eating habits and balanced nutrition. Yes, there are many effective programs, but in the course of learning about health, fitness, nutrition, and exercise, I learned things about *me.* I came to realize that while the program at UAMS is terrific, some people have tried it and quit. Still others have used different methods and succeeded where I failed. Why?

I have become more convinced than ever that while there are numerous outstanding weight loss plans, a person focused only on losing weight is likely doomed to failure. Been there, done that, and I have a closetful of XXL T-shirts to prove it!

I have friends and family members who have lost weight using Atkins, Weight Watchers, South Beach, Sugar Busters, Jenny Craig, and others. If these methods work for you, congratulations and go for it! This book won't condemn anyone's method. My experience is that most people fail not because their *method* fails them, but because their *motivation* fails them. The challenge is not so much to change your actions on a temporary basis but rather to change your attitudes on a permanent basis.

I'm going to share with you "12 STOPs" I consider critical to motivating your *mind* so your *method* will work–to making clear that the goal is not weight loss but health and fitness. *You can do it* and experience a permanent change in lifestyle.

Okay, I know you're tempted to close the book and head for the kitchen and grab a bag of potato chips while you contemplate whether you should give this a try. You may even be thinking, *It's fine that it worked for him, but it won't work for me.*

I would have thought the same thing because I am by nature a skeptic, but I can now share some changes I experienced that I never thought were possible. I was never, ever a "gym rat" who worked out, stayed fit, and took care of myself–not even during times of my life when I wasn't excessively overweight. I spent the first forty-eight years of my life doing almost everything possible to model bad habits. At times, I believe that the transformation I've experienced is nothing short of miraculous. What I will share with you will be so simple, you'll wonder why you haven't already heard it. Maybe because many "health" books are written by people who have lived healthy lives, and people like that assume everyone else is mostly just like them and simply needs some good recipes, a few platitudes, and a calorie counter.

The simple yet profound lessons you're about to discover are lessons I learned by asking myself and others *why* questions more than *what* questions. All along the journey I had "Aha!" moments. When I'd tell friends about principles I was putting into practice, the response would be, "Wow, I never thought of that." Or "That's really profound–you ought to write that stuff down and put it in a book." When I gave the first draft of the manuscript to some friends to determine if it was really useful, the reactions were stunning. One friend had battled bulimia as a teenager and came to me in tears, saying, "I wish I'd had this book when I was seventeen." I didn't even anticipate its application for anything other than helping out middle-aged fat guys!

I knew things in my life had changed when, upon checking into a hotel, my first order of business was finding out when the fitness center opened rather than what was offered on the room service menu and how late the kitchen was open. Be assured that I'm not starving. I eat a wide variety of wonderful, delicious foods, most of which I've enjoyed all my life, and I do not feel the least bit deprived.

Amazingly, I actually enjoy the food I eat more than ever.

What do you have to lose? Some weight? Maybe a little bit of time. But most important, you might want to lose some of those bad habits that are keeping you from successfully losing weight and getting on the path to forever fitness. So let's get started—or maybe I should say:

Let's get STOPped!

DEAR GOVERNOR,

I commend you for what you have done for your state but more im-
portantly what you have done for your own health. I believe that
your life experience has meant a great deal for your state and country
as well. After reading your story, I was influenced to do something
about my weight problem since I, like you, was also diagnosed with
diabetes shortly after my father passed away in 1977.

Pennsylvania

Before You Begin

Chances are your doctor has been telling you for a long time that you need to lose weight. Every time you go to see him or her, regardless of the purpose of the visit, you are likely to be reminded that you are overweight and need to do something about it. He probably suggests "diet and exercise," and you smile, nod in agreement, then walk out of the office, stop for ice cream on the way home, and continue to do exactly what you have been doing.

This time, shock him. Go to him and tell him you really are serious about weight loss and fitness. Ask him to test all the basics: blood sugar, blood pressure, A1C hemoglobin, cholesterol levels. You need to establish a baseline of where you are in your personal health, so you will have something to compare yourself with over the coming months. Let your focus be not so much on how many pounds you lose but on achieving true fitness and health. Focus on lowering your blood pressure, blood sugar, cholesterol levels, and most notably that sense of "forever fatigue" and lethargy that you have learned to live with, and even overcome, but which robs you of a sense of exuberance and excitement each day.

Decide what method you will use as your weight loss vehicle. Your doctor may have a regimen for you.

While participating in the National Summit on Obesity, sponsored by TIME magazine and ABC News in June 2004 in Williamsburg, Virginia, I was intrigued by a panel consisting of the creators of many of the most popular diet plans on the market. There were some common denominators in the approaches touted by the various authors and doctors who'd originated some of the best-known and most widely marketed diet plans.

If you're looking for a "secret" to successful weight loss, there isn't one. Despite the many claims of infomercials on television pushing "miracle" pills, formulas, and exercise devices that supposedly let you eat anything you want, all you want, and as often as you want, the truth is that weight loss comes back to this simple truth—fewer calories *in* (consumption) and more calories *out* (exercise). Even though my doctors told me "diet and exercise" for years, I kept hoping that there really would be a product developed that would let me take an easier path. I dreamed of unlimited portions of unlimited foods and the only exercise necessary being an extra trip to the buffet or the lifting of a fork, but there is no such path to health. Such is the path to disaster.

Because I wouldn't want to risk getting charged with practicing medicine without a license, I will not try to give you a medical prescription for your method. I will, however, ask—in fact, *demand*—that for the *next twelve days* you will stick to the plan with a religious zeal. During these initial twelve days there will be no cheating whatsoever—*none*! The reason for this is twofold. First, you need to prove to yourself that you can do it. More important, though, your body needs to literally detox. After these all-important first twelve days, you will begin to experience a self-perpetuating motivation, and you'll begin to lose those insatiable cravings that helped engineer your downfall in previous attempts.

I'm asked several times a day, "What kind of food do you eat?" As I eat meals at banquets or public functions, people come up and say, "I just wanted to see what *you* are eating." The program I worked with at the University of Arkansas for Medical Sciences (UAMS) was helpful because it was divided into three phases. The first was an intense and somewhat dramatic change of eating habits that eliminated sugar and high-glycemic-index foods like potatoes and pasta, focusing instead on prepared soups and drinks that satisfied my hunger and nutritional needs, and furthered a sense of significant departure from my typical routine. It worked for me because I didn't have to think, plan, or fret about what I could or couldn't eat. I needed that intense "break-away" from having to choose my food until I changed *me* enough to make smart choices. You will reach several plateaus as you move toward regaining your health, but this is not a temporary diet to lose your big balloon of a belly. Temporary diets only lead to temporary weight loss–this is changing your life.

I wrote this book for people like me who want to be "recovering foodaholics." I hope to offer help and hope to you if, like me, you have often found yourself finishing lunch and planning dinner. Or if you've ever driven up and down a busy boulevard having a hard time deciding where to stop for food, not because you were unable to find something appealing, but because you found *everything* appealing, and ended up stopping at more than one of the places you saw!

For years, I tried the "see-food" diet–I would *see* food, I'd want to eat it, and I often did. My appetite consumed me as much as I consumed food. I was addicted to the notion that any good food was even better when consumed in mass quantities, and loved menus that featured items labeled *jumbo, extra large, supersize, king-cut* . . . I wondered if I would ever have control of my appetite instead of my appetite having control of me. As I retrained and reconditioned my metabolism and began to understand how certain foods not only made me fat but also triggered a more aggressive appetite, I finally experienced the kind of breakthrough that enabled me to make these changes as a lifestyle and not merely a limitation of desires.

This book is not intended to *supplant* your favorite diet plan or book, but to *supplement* it. The 12 STOPs don't *compete* with a plan you like; they are designed to *complete* the plan with insights into how to move from a "program" to permanent changes in your health and fitness.

Because I'm often asked to simply list some fundamental foods to eat or to avoid, let me give you the "12 STOPs of Food Choices" that are fairly common to every weight loss or fitness plan you will encounter.

1. **STOP consuming trans fats or TFA (trans-fatty acid).**
   If it reads "partially hydrogenated vegetable oil" on the label, consider eating the package and throwing away the food! By 2006, federal law will require food labels to list the amount of trans fats in a food. That will help you steer clear of them.

2. **STOP avoiding your fruits and vegetables!**
   The National Cancer Institute has a simple slogan: *5 A Day.* This is a reminder to eat *at least* five

servings of fruits and vegetables every day. That's a minimum! Eat them as close to the way God made them as possible—don't overcook them or smother them with sauces and butter. They really do taste great!

3. **STOP eating refined sugar.**
That includes "hidden sugar" such as the high-fructose corn syrup found in many foods.

4. **STOP eating highly processed foods.**
Eat things that your body actually gets to digest—that's what it was designed to do! If you eat highly processed foods, you eat food that a machine has digested for you. These give you more empty calories than they do nutrition.

5. **STOP large portions.**
A portion about the size of your fist is a good rule of thumb (or rule of fist?). As hard a habit as it is to break, do *not* order the supersize version unless you plan to share it with at least two other people at your table!

6. **STOP skipping meals.**
Skipping meals is *not* a means of losing weight, but rather a way to gain it. The body thinks you're going to starve it, so it slows down your metabolism. It is especially critical never to skip breakfast. I did this for years to "lose weight" and ended up gaining the weight of a Saint Bernard!

7. STOP ignoring calories.

Watch your total calorie consumption, and be sure to eat two thousand calories or less per day.

8. STOP eating only three meals a day.

That's right—eat smaller portions five or six times a day rather than three larger meals. Spacing out the food intake helps keep you from feeling "starved" at mealtime and keeps you satisfied longer without gorging yourself. Eat a good breakfast, then have a light snack midmorning, a light lunch, another light snack midafternoon (fruit, nuts perhaps), a sensible dinner, and—if your dinner is early and you're up late—perhaps another *very* light snack in the evening.

9. STOP dehydration.

Drink *lots* of water—at least eight glasses (at least eight ounces each) per day. Your urine should be clear (and if you drink the amount of water you should, you'll have plenty of opportunities to check!).

10. STOP eating fried foods.

'Nuff said!

11. STOP eating high-glycemic-index foods.

In addition to avoiding sugar like you would avoid ingesting rat poison, stay away from the high-glycemic-index foods such as starchy vegetables (potatoes, for example), white bread, and so on.

12. STOP depriving yourself of good grains.
You should eat whole-grain breads, cereals, and pastas, but be aware that whole grain isn't the same as "wheat bread," which may be overly processed and would fall into the category of high-glycemic-index foods. It might be necessary to shop at a natural food store, where the bread or pasta is made from whole grains and not from bleached, enriched, or processed flour.

These are simple yet fundamental dos and don'ts that can give you a quick-start guide to healthy and pleasurable eating. However, I will say repeatedly (repetition is the mother of all learning!) that your goal is not just "losing fat," but "gaining fitness." One can be done in a few months—the other takes a lifetime.

I want you to do more than change your *figure*—I want you to help you change your *future*!

As you begin the first steps of this journey, let me be among the first to congratulate you for taking control of an area of your life that has been out of control for a long time.

DEAR GOVERNOR,

I know you hear this over and over, but you are a true inspiration for those who think they can't accomplish something. Most people don't realize it just takes one foot in front of the other to make it to the finish line and succeed.

Pediatrician, Arkansas

STOP 1

STOP Procrastinating

It has been said that "the road to hell is paved with good intentions," but unquestionably the road to *obesity* is paved with procrastination.

Remember the closing scene in the classic movie *Gone With the Wind*? Ever-so-thin Scarlett O'Hara declares, "I'll think about it tomorrow. After all, tomorrow is another day." We believe we can always start getting healthy tomorrow.

Most of us who have battled with weight issues can perhaps identify more readily with another of Scarlett O'Hara's memorable scenes—the one where she is digging up potatoes and saying, "I'll never be hungry again!" Indeed, we wouldn't be just digging up the potatoes but also eating them, preferably fried. Our goal is never to be hungry again!

One of the main reasons most of us yearn to get fit but never do is because we fail to STOP PROCRASTINATING. It is simply easier to plan on health and fitness but never to do it, by marking our intentions with a definite date in the future that we never seem to keep:

"I'm going to start my new diet right after the holidays."

"I'm going to get some of this weight off in time for summer."

"I'm getting ready to get back into a fitness routine so I'll look good for my daughter's wedding."

You've heard it *all* before. Heck, you've *said* it all before! The problem is most of us make sure that whenever it is we're going to start our new regimen, one thing's for sure—it *won't* be today.

A number of years ago, I produced some TV documentaries in Guatemala. Whenever I'd ask my local guide or translator when we'd have certain materials, he'd say, "*Mañana.*" I thought that meant "tomorrow." I'd ask the same question the next day and get the same answer—"*Mañana.*" I grew frustrated with the delays and angry that the promises were never kept. Finally one of the locals explained to me, "*Mañana* doesn't mean 'tomorrow'—it means 'not today.'"

Are you on the *mañana* diet? There is a good likelihood that if you procrastinate about health and fitness, you procrastinate about other things as well. Finally getting control of this unwieldy area of your life could mean a dramatic new opportunity to create personal discipline that extends far beyond your (hopefully shrinking) waistline.

If anyone has ever had an excuse for putting off a healthy lifestyle, I would claim that *my* excuse was as good as any could be. As a sitting governor, my life is about as complicated as anyone's, and the schedule I keep is more challenging than most people will ever comprehend. Several full-time employees in my office do nothing but work on scheduling my every waking moment—sometimes scheduling those moments when I'm not even awake! We receive literally hundreds of invitations for me to be a part of events ranging from ribbon cuttings to royal visits, and without a doubt this is the most challenging part of my job. Most of the places I go and things I do are reactions to other people's agendas and priorities. When people ask, "How do you find time to exercise?" I respond, "I don't *find* the time, I *make* the time!" If you wait until you "find" time, you will *never*–hear me–*never* find it. You must *make* time for taking care of your body just as you make time to go to work, to shower, to eat, or to take in a movie.

There are also a tremendous number of disruptions to my schedule that I must be prepared for: special legislative sessions; natural disasters (frankly, sometimes it's difficult to tell the difference between a legislative session and a tornado); budget crises; managing more than fifty cabinet-level agencies; being responsible for more than 320 boards, agencies, and commissions; and managing fifty thousand employees, not to mention policies that touch issues ranging from police to prisons, education, health care, highways, environment, employment, and taxes.

Despite constant pleadings from my family, close friends, and doctor, I could always articulate a good reason why "this would not be a good time to make changes in my eating or exercise habits." *Mañana!*

On several occasions, I even made specific plans to do something about my ever-expanding girth. But I prepared for the day by trying to eat my way through all the various stored junk foods I had accumulated, convincing myself it would be improper to let those good foods go to waste!

Putting a date on the calendar several weeks ahead, I would proceed to munch my way through closets or cabinets where a good stock of potato chips, candy, and other delicious items had been carefully hoarded for just such an occasion. Of course, by the time I had finished devouring all those items, the ever-vigilant staff at the Governor's Mansion would see to it that the supplies were replenished. By then I had arranged a whole new list of reasons to put off the project for another month or more. *Mañana!*

Getting past an upcoming event was always one of my favorite excuses. "I'll start eating right as soon as Thanksgiving and Christmas are over." Oh, sure! Then comes the Super Bowl—"No use starting a diet until at least then!" Of course, by then it's another occasion, then another, then another, and then another. Between big holidays, birthdays, and special events such as church feasts and political fish-fry rallies, I could always find reasons to wait "one more week." I even became good at celebrating holidays for other people. How many Baptists do you know who observe all the Jewish feasts?

I also rationalized that as long as the cupboards were filled with expensive—albeit unhealthy—foods, it would be a shame to waste them. "I'll start eating right as soon as we finish off all this junk food once and for all." (Of course, we always found a way to replace that food with more just like it!)

Looking ahead to travel opportunities provided another great excuse. "I'll be in New Orleans in two weeks, and I won't be able to go there and not enjoy the wonderful Creole and Cajun foods. Next month, I'll be in Chicago, and what would a trip to Chicago be without Chicago-style pizza? And then there's the cruise we're going to take for our anniversary, and I'd be crazy not to enjoy all those midnight buffets!"

My wife carefully reminded me of a promise I had made to her on my fortieth birthday. In August 1995, I'd told Janet that I was getting to the age where I was increasingly vulnerable to a heart attack given the high stress I experienced on the job, genetic factors, and my sedentary lifestyle. I told her one of the key things to help me maintain my health would be a new bass boat, which would let me more effectively pursue a form of recreation that I found relaxing and therapeutic—bass fishing. For several months I regaled her with the virtues of my owning a new bass boat, most notably that its cost would certainly be much less than the cost of a heart attack. Amazingly, she believed it, and on my fortieth birthday she gave me a brand-new, fully equipped Bass Cat fishing boat with a 225-horsepower Mercury outboard motor.

Unfortunately, it would be several years before I would finally live up to my part of the deal by taking better care of myself.

I will be the first to admit that changing a lifetime of bad habits isn't easy. But it won't be any easier tomorrow, next week, next year, or after one of those artificial milestones such as a graduation or special birthday. There are four basic principles that are essential to being able to STOP PROCRASTINATING:

1. *Set* a very specific and definite start time for your program within the next two weeks.
2. *Share* your start date with several trusted friends, family members, and perhaps your doctor.
3. *Start!* After you set it and share it, start it! Don't let *anything* keep you from this very important and hopefully life-changing appointment.
4. *Stick* to it!

Even more difficult than setting a very specific time to start changing your eating habits is to stop procrastinating your personal exercise routine. I will deal with the importance of physical activity a little later. But for now let me focus on how important it is to stop putting off *some kind* of activity.

The easiest thing in the world for me was to justify exercising *tomorrow* rather than *today*. One of the most stressful aspects of my job is that it's never finished, no matter how many papers I sign, speeches I make, appointments I keep, or events I attend. There are multitudes more looming on the horizon. I enjoy cooking as a hobby, largely because the preparation of a meal has a very definite point of beginning and it has a point of completion, the results are obvious and immediate, and there is the potential of gratification when the recipe turns out well. Doing anything that draws to a conclusion and offers closure and finality is quite rewarding. So on any given day, when I was tempted to begin an exercise regime, I could always remind myself of other things yet undone on my "to-do" list and justify procrastinating an exercise routine until at least tomorrow.

One of my most thrilling accomplishments in my quest for regained health occurred during the first holiday season when I was taking care of myself and actually *lost* weight instead of *gaining* it for possibly the first time in my life. I was determined I would not ruin my many months of hard work to get fit by indulging in all the holiday treats that would inevitably be shoved at me and available around the clock. I knew it would be one of the great tests of whether I was simply going through a "phase" or if this was a serious change of lifestyle. Please understand that I define the *holiday season* as that period between Thanksgiving and the Super Bowl. I'm talking Thanksgiving, the days leading up to and through Christmas, and New Year's (with its vast amount of football watching and endless eating). My holiday season doesn't end until after Super Bowl weekend, which is best described as an event in which twenty-two athletes on a field who are desperate for rest are watched by seventy thousand in a stadium and millions more at home who are desperate for exercise!

More amazing than my ability to get through this two-month

period without cheating and actually losing weight instead of gaining was the fact that I never really wanted to get off the wagon. Traditionally, "Christmas at the Capitol," in the governor's office as well as at the Governor's Mansion, is a never-ending series of holiday events, all of which involve enormous amounts of delicious but decidedly fattening foods. Numerous deliveries are made daily to the office and mansion with holiday treats ranging from fruitcakes to cookies, candies, pies, glazed nuts, and fudge. Because of the STOPs I had made and the steps I had taken, for the first time in my life I not only was able to resist the temptation to indulge in those foods but actually got more pleasure from saying "no thank you" than I would have received from eating.

As you can imagine, there is an extraordinary level of satisfaction from having people notice the improved appearance of personal fitness. There's not a day that goes by in which I'm not approached by someone who says, "You look amazing." I'm thrilled, but also know it means that before I must have really looked awful!

Frank Broyles is the athletic director and former head football coach of the University of Arkansas Razorbacks. He coached the 1964 Razorbacks team to the national championship and continues to serve as athletic director even though he is now in his seventies. He is still a remarkably fit man and a role model for living an active healthy life. I appeared with Coach Broyles at an event in Fayetteville in late 2003. It had been several months since he had seen me. In that period of time, I had dropped an extraordinary amount of weight, and he was quite effusive in congratulating me and commending me for my changes in lifestyle. He said something to me that day that I thought was very profound. I've used it again and again on days when I thought that maybe I should indulge myself in some of the guilty pleasures of cheesecake, pecan pie, or mashed potatoes with gravy. He said, "Governor, I found years ago that nothing ever tastes as good as it feels to be thin."

How true that is! As someone who has tried almost every kind of delicious food to be found on earth, I have to say that I can affirm Coach Broyles's statement. Nothing does taste as good as it feels to be thin, or–as I would put it–"Nothing tastes as good as it feels to be healthy."

So STOP number one on the road to forever fitness is

STOP PROCRASTINATING–DO IT NOW!

DEAR GOVERNOR,

I have been a resident of this state for the past 15 years of my life. I don't pay much attention to politics, but I can't keep quiet any longer. I want to congratulate you on your weight loss and commend you on all the things you have done on obesity issues. I myself have been obese all my life. Actually, I was severe morbidly obese. Now I am just obese. I didn't know you had lost weight until I started losing mine. I was a prisoner in my bedroom when I wasn't at work. I know that is a little more information than you probably want, but I just felt I had to tell you. Obesity has always been a personal problem, and I am so glad you have brought it even more to the public's attention. I wish there were more I could do.

You have always been this person that I heard about on the news or read about in the paper, but never had anything in common with. I guess I [can say] now that we are both "losers." Weight losers! This is one situation where I'm glad to be a loser. I don't agree with everything you have done in office, but I can tell you that I'm 110% behind you on weight issues.

Arkansas

STOP 2

STOP Making Excuses

If I'd received a dime for every excuse I ever gave for not get-ting adequate exercise or eating properly, I could have made a very comfortable living. But if you want to experience the kind of forever fitness that changes the way you feel and look, it becomes very important to STOP.

Let me list some of my excuses. Have a look and see if they are similar to the ones you've used. Perhaps you will even have some that I haven't thought of. (Please don't send them to me–I don't need any more in my repertoire!) I mentioned some of these in the introduction, but let's talk some more about those ex-cuses that are so easy to make.

1. **I'm genetically predisposed toward being overweight.**
   There is no doubt some truth to the idea that certain traits or characteristics are indeed genetic. Some of us are predisposed toward diabetes, heart

disease, or even alcoholism, but that is a flimsy excuse for not taking care of ourselves. In fact, if we know we are genetically predisposed toward a certain characteristic, we should work even harder to avoid its consequences. As I have mentioned, weight has been a problem in my family for generations as best I can tell. I've often said that a Huckabee family reunion at an all-you-can-eat buffet could put the place out of business in one day! My own parents, who are now both deceased, were diabetic and had myriad health issues, mostly related to overeating, eating foods high in calories and low in nutrition, and failing to get adequate exercise.

My father suffered a heart attack and had coronary bypass surgery in his early sixties. My mother had surgery to unclog her femoral arteries and later experienced a debilitating aneurism and stroke that led to a long and very difficult struggle until her death. Two of my grandparents were also diabetic. If there is such a thing as genetic disposition toward obesity and poor health, I certainly was justified in claiming it. But it was *my choices,* not just my genetics, that put me in a position of crisis.

2. **I'm large-boned.**
This has to be one of my all-time favorites! What this means, no one seems to know, other than that it's an excuse for being larger than we're supposed

to be. We can claim that we have very little skin or fat surrounding these enormous bones that we supposedly have inherited. Of course, unless we've had a complete skeletal X-ray, I'm not sure how we determine that our over-the-top weight is the result of bone density . . . but it sure sounds more acceptable to say "I'm large-boned" than it does to say "I consume the dietary needs of six people" or "I eat the same amount of food as a medium-size village in Ethiopia."

3. **It's cultural.**

   I have already confessed to the impact and effect my Southern roots have had on my habits of diet and exercise, but most cultures can be used as a basis or excuse not to eat properly or exercise. My friends in Wisconsin can talk about their civic duty to consume massive amounts of dairy products and defer exercise to those few months a year when it's not snowing outside. Folks in Philadelphia can claim that in their culture, the classic cheese steak sandwich is as much a staple food as is Southern-fried catfish in Mississippi or heavily marbled beef in Texas. Large quantities of corn in Nebraska, extra helpings of smoked ham in Iowa, or even a trayful of milk- and sugar-laden lattes from Seattle are regional excuses. The reality is that while culture is assuredly an influence and at times a dominating one, we ultimately do what we do because we *choose* to do it.

4. **I don't have time to exercise, and certainly don't have time for planning what I eat.**

   Actually, each of us has the same amount of time as everyone else. We all have 168 hours a week no matter what our race, gender, ethnic background, or religion might be. It's not how much time we have, but how we allocate our time that determines whether or not we will schedule exercise and whether or not we will make time to eat right. We either believe good habits will keep us alive or we ignore them because somehow we think that watching an extra episode of *Jeopardy!* is worth more to us than shopping for the ingredients of a fresh salad (which we know would be healthier than a can of fat-filled goo disguised as a meal that will only clog our arteries). Remember what I said in the last chapter. You will never *find* the time—you *make* the time!

5. **I've tried every diet before, and none has worked.**

   This was one of my favorite excuses for quite some time. I actually successfully followed the Atkins diet as a teenager. Indeed, over the years I've been on about every type of diet imaginable, from low-fat to all-protein to low-carb to diets that consisted mostly of cabbage soup or bananas. I even tried fen-phen and liquid-only diets. All of them worked to a degree, but the problem was I did not make a substantial lifestyle change and viewed the diet as simply a temporary measure to lose weight rather than as a catalyst for making permanent changes to what I ate, when I ate it, how much I ate, and what kind of activity I participated in. One of the fundamental differences this time is that I never set out to lose a specific amount of weight. When people asked, "How much are you trying to lose?" I would tell them I did not have a *weight* goal but rather a *health and fitness* goal. Even if you've tried every diet imaginable, try something different this time. Instead of considering yourself on a diet, consider yourself on a *life mission* to adjust your eating habits and accept the fact that you cannot succeed at this unless you are willing to sustain it for your lifetime. Even if you adopt a method of weight loss that features an initial phase of excluding a certain type of food, or eating only certain things, or using meal replacements such as protein shakes or what have you, make sure you realize that in the long term, you have to learn how to eat rationally and nutritionally.

6. **Health plans are just too expensive!**
   Funerals are expensive, too, especially when you have to hire extra people to lift your casket! The program for the weight loss phase that I participated in at the University of Arkansas for Medical Sciences (UAMS) was somewhat expensive, but by reversing some health issues I was able to discontinue taking several prescribed medications. The savings from those monthly medications is more than making up for my cost of participating in the program. As it turned out, the

biggest expense I encountered with this health routine was the cost of altering and eventually replacing virtually everything in my wardrobe! By the time I got some things back from the alteration shop, they were already too large. It got to the point at which I found that my clothes could not be altered anymore. For those who have never experienced this, just be aware that when your front pockets become your back pockets and your back pockets join together, it's probably time to get a new pair of pants!

If you continue to believe it's simply too expensive to get healthy, think about the cost of being unhealthy. Your insurance policy costs more. Your medical bills are substantially more, and your pharmacy bills are staggering. You pay more for big-size clothing, and your choices are far more limited. If trends continue, you might even have to start paying for an additional airline seat or theater seat. You don't have to enroll in an expensive club or clinic to develop healthy habits. But you do have to STOP MAKING EXCUSES.

Maybe you have tried and failed and tried and failed and tried and failed and you are wondering—*Why keep trying?* Because maybe you simply haven't tried enough!

When you learned to ride a bike as a child, you didn't immediately get up on the two wheels and ride. Most likely you tried to get on the bicycle but fell and skinned your knees. But you tried again and then again and then again until you finally got the hang of it.

My daughter, Sarah, the youngest of our three children, recently graduated from college, and she now works in Washington, DC. When she was just a few months old, she decided one day that she would take her first steps walking. She had spent the first months of her life observing the art of walking through her father, mother, and two older brothers, and it was obvious that walking was a great improvement over rolling and crawling. She seemed quite determined to take her first steps and join the rest of the family in walking where she needed to go. I will never forget the day she made her first attempt. She crawled over to a little table in our family den, pulled herself up, and let go for what she anticipated would be the first of many steps. Instead of scooting across the floor in an upright position, she tumbled forward and landed flat on her face. I could see in her eyes that it was quite a disappointing moment for her.

She then crawled over to the corner of the room, sat up, and announced to all of us in a clear, firm voice, "Well, I tried walking and it just didn't work for me. While I realize it works for you, Mom, John Mark, and David, you can clearly see that after months of anticipating and preparing and even studying for this moment, I have attempted to walk and have failed. Because I tried to walk and have been unsuccessful in my attempt, I suppose I will have to trust and depend on you and others in the family to carry me wherever I go for the rest of my life."

Of course Sarah didn't do that or say that! She did pull herself up to the little table and attempt to start walking. She did fall flat on her face. But instead of quitting, she went right back to the same table and stood again and tried again. She repeated this over and over until she finally was so exhausted that she lay on the floor and went to sleep. Later she tried again and fell, and again and fell, and again and fell, and continued until she was able to take a few small steps. It wasn't long before she was taking many steps across the floor and then around the house and then the neighborhood. Now it's difficult to keep up with her!

Very few musicians sit at the keyboard of a piano for the first time and play a masterpiece. I've been playing the guitar since I was eleven years old, and I can remember how painful it was in those early days when my fingers came close to bleeding from hours upon hours of practice. I now play in my own rock-and-roll band made up mostly of governor's office staff and some friends. We call ourselves "Capitol Offense" and are having the time of our lives as a bunch of middle-aged people playing classic rock and roll and living the dream of musicians.

Since I'm the only sitting governor in America with his own rock band, we get invited to some pretty good gigs. We've opened arena concerts for Willie Nelson, the Charlie Daniels Band, Grand Funk Railroad, Dionne Warwick, Percy Sledge, .38 Special, and others. We have played at inaugural parties for President Bush, conferences for the Southern Governors' Association and Council of State Governments, the Education Commission of the States, and a host of charity events. In New York, we even played an outdoor concert hosted by Governor George Pataki during the 2004 Republican National Convention.

An extraordinary amount of pleasure can be derived from playing a musical instrumental and hearing the applause of several thousand people in an audience. But in the early days when I first plunked around on the inexpensive electric guitar that my parents got me for Christmas in 1966 from the J. C. Penney catalog, I would have found it hard to believe that I would someday be playing with ease with professional musicians and recording artists.

A few years back when Grand Funk Railroad was in Little

Rock playing a reunion tour, I was asked to sit in with them during a sound check and play bass while they rehearsed. As I stood there watching guitarist and vocalist Mark Farner just a few feet away playing guitar and singing, it occurred to me that a group that I'd idolized as a teenager was playing one of their hit songs and here I was in the middle of it, belting out bass notes on "Some Kind of Wonderful." In 2004, one of the great country bands of all time, Alabama, came to Little Rock as part of their farewell tour. We hosted a lunch for the legendary musicians and artists. I was in heaven! That night, they invited me to the stage to play bass with them on their hit "I'm in a Hurry." Later, a friend of mine with whom I once played in a garage band in high school asked how I was able to play with Grand Funk Railroad, Alabama, or country singer Collin Raye. My first response was, "Practice man, practice." Truthfully, of course, it had more to do with being governor than it did with being good, but whether it's sports, music, or exercising and eating right, it never works to make the excuse "I've tried it and it didn't work." So STOP number two is one that becomes all-important:

STOP MAKING EXCUSES.

DEAR GOVERNOR,

I received this article [about your weight loss] from my sister last week from the Baltimore newspaper. I thought to myself, Another article about me having diabetes. *I was diagnosed two years ago this month with type II. It scared me to death and I was very upset that I had gotten this way. How could I have done that? My doctor is very strict but I need someone like that who is in my face. He sent me to a six-week class on diabetes. I fought with him about not going and cried a lot. When I got there I was the only one who had not had a heart attack or lost a limb, etc. That even made me want to fight more. I now walk one hour every day and have lost 40 lbs. My doctor still wants me to lose more and I will continue with a healthy lifestyle for the rest of my life because I'm still scared. After I had read your article I started reading it over and over again and even cried over it because my goal in life is to get off medicine forever. In your article I read that you do recumbent bike. I knew I had one in the basement but had never used it. Surprised by that? Well, I did it for the first time tonight, and I thought that if you can do [it] so could I. I did ride it for 20 minutes and will start every night after my hour walk. Hopefully I will finish my weight goal even sooner. Maybe when I go back to the doctor in October things will start looking even better than they had. I do want you to know that I was glad my sister did send me this article and how much you have inspired me. I even gave the article to my doctor and a co-worker. I will also be doing the Diabetes Association Charity Walk in Sept. Thanks again for giving me some help along the way and knowing when I'm down I will take out your article. Stay healthy!*

Missouri

STOP 3

STOP Sitting on the Couch

During the first thirty years of my adult life, I tried at various times to diet and lose weight, and on a few occasions I attempted to start an exercise program. I inevitably failed at both. What I hadn't really tried to do was make realistic and reachable efforts at both of them at the same time. I had to develop a more comprehensive approach to health, as opposed to simply trying to get rid of some excess pounds within a specific time frame and for a specific purpose.

As difficult as it was to occasionally change my eating habits during a diet, it was easy compared with attempting an exercise program. While I like sports and enjoyed participating in them as a small child, by the time I got to junior high school it became pretty apparent to me that I probably would never be quarterbacking the Dallas Cowboys to a Super Bowl victory; nor would I be named MVP in the NBA. Exercise for me was more than difficult—it was virtually impossible. It was easy to find things to do that were more urgent and on which other people were depending. I could always rationalize that exercise was selfish because it was only benefiting me, but my work was benefiting others and therefore took precedence. Frankly, no one has been more surprised than me to discover that I not only tolerate daily exercise but am almost fanatical about it. On days when my schedule calls for earlier-than-normal activities, instead of skipping my morning exercise routine, I simply set my alarm clock earlier and roust myself out of bed as early as three thirty in the morning in order to get in my walking, running, recumbent-bike-riding, or weight-lifting routine.

I cannot completely describe just how contemptuous I was of exercise and those who engaged in it regularly. I used to say, "What's the point of going jogging if, while you're trotting down the road, you're run over by a large truck?" Maybe you're as good as I was about finding reasons to not exercise, but you *can* turn your life around. To do so, you must make the conscious decision to STOP SITTING ON THE COUCH.

Most people fail at an exercise routine because they start out doing more than is reasonable or realistic. Let me suggest what worked for me. I hope it will work for you.

It's really important to have a visit with your doctor before embarking on a program to change your eating habits dramatically or start exercising. Be sure you tell him or her what you are attempting to do and why you are there. Make a list of questions to ask:

- What are the limits of physical activity I should do?
- Are my feet, ankles, knees, hips, and so on, in good shape for walking?
- How's my blood pressure? Blood sugar? Cholesterol?
- Will eating (or not eating) certain things be a problem and potentially aggravate my system?

If your doctor doesn't want to really help you in this and acts as if she's only interested in treating your diseases and not preventing them, then a word of advice—*Get a new doctor!* I'm not kidding! You *must* have a doctor who would rather see you get healthy and not need her so often, not one who looks at you like a lab rat to be treated with an ever-changing array of expensive drugs and procedures designed to confront your symptoms, but not help you change your lifestyle. I've been amazed at how much less I even get the sniffles since getting healthy, and my chronic problems with upper respiratory illnesses are few and far between. Try to remember that your job is not to contract the "disease of the month" so your doctor will have something to do.

Visit with your doctor. Ask questions. Get advice. Then get busy!

If you are tremendously overweight, your doctor may advise you (as mine did) to lose at least some weight before attempting any exercise routine. Your weight can have a huge impact on your ability to safely to put into motion even the simplest of routines, such as walking.

Set aside only twelve minutes per day at the outset—not a minute more, unless you are already in the habit of exercising. Limit yourself to twelve and only twelve minutes. Most people fail in an exercise routine because they start at an activity level that is too intense or for a time period that they cannot maintain. As you develop healthy habits, you will make the decision to increase the time and rigor of the activity, but the key is to be consistent in exercising at least twelve minutes.

Make your exercise routine simple and inexpensive. I strongly suggest that you not rush out and join a health club or fitness center or buy a gym membership just yet. Spend your twelve minutes exercising—not driving to and from the gym! You would likely feel silly driving fifteen or twenty minutes to a gym, exercising for twelve minutes, and then driving fifteen or twenty minutes back home. If you join a gym, chances are you will want to work with a trainer, who will probably start you on far more rigorous exercise than you are physically or mentally capable of handling at the outset. There will perhaps come a time when you will seek out the services of a professional, or maybe join a gym or health club, but now is not necessarily that time. The goal right now is stopping the bad habits.

To do that, you need to focus on the things that will truly help adjust your life in the simplest and least expensive way possible.

To start, get up fifteen to twenty minutes earlier than you did yesterday so that you don't have to squeeze these twelve minutes of exercise into your already crowded schedule. If you're convinced that you're rushed, you'll do what I inevitably did in the past and say, "I'll exercise tomorrow, but today I'm really in a hurry and I just don't have the time." It is true that you probably don't have time unless you *make the time* by scheduling your twelve minutes of exercise just as you'd schedule a bath, breakfast, or putting on your clothes. Surely you allow time for those activities. You need to wake up fifteen to twenty minutes earlier so that you will have more than the twelve minutes you'll need for the exercise routine you choose.

You may already have a closetful of exercise equipment you've bought at various times in your life when you were determined to get fit but failed. If any of this gear appeals to you now, use it. But if you absolutely hated it before, it is doubtful you will wake up one day and find yourself thrilled with utilizing some piece of fabulous fitness equipment you ordered from a television infomercial. I suggest you start by doing something that requires no additional money and no special equipment and can be done virtually wherever you are: Get out and walk. Taking a twelve-minute walk a day may not seem like a tremendous stretch of your abilities, but if you have done nothing but sit on a couch for years, even twelve minutes of walking a day will help get you started on some good habits and, more important, stop the bad ones. Walking is good exercise because it's simple, requires no training, and can be carried out almost regardless of weather or other conditions.

I like starting the day with exercise, because it's before I am likely to receive telephone calls, have interruptions, or start thinking of reasons why I don't have time. While I've always been an early riser, I now get up most mornings at about 4:30 AM to get a good start on the day. It may not be necessary for you to get up at 4:30 AM of course; depending on your own body clock, waking up at 8:00 AM may be a true challenge for you.

Some of my friends are night people and find that a walk or exercise just before bedtime is perfect for them, while others, including some on my staff, use their lunch hour to get in a walk or even a run and feel that it gives them a great midday boost and helps them avoid the midafternoon sluggishness so commonly experienced.

We aren't all wired the same, so while getting up at four thirty works for me, such a time might be as appealing or practical to you as having the hair burned off your head instead of simply getting a haircut. Do what works for you. The key is to *do something*!

In the early stages, simply adjust your routine by fifteen to twenty minutes and walk according to the clock, focusing on twelve minutes as opposed to a particular distance. Use your walking time to plan your day, to think about why your health is important to you, to review the various STOPs you need to adhere to in order to be successful, and what you will and will not eat that day. In the early stages, it's probably best that you walk alone. There is a good chance that if you walk with others, they will want to walk longer than twelve minutes—which may be more than you can handle at first. Or you might end up waiting on them to join you, which means you'll resent the extra time you've devoted when you only committed to twelve minutes.

At first, don't worry about how fast you walk or how far. Remember, your goal is stopping bad habits and starting good ones—not winning first prize. Initially, I found that twelve minutes of exercise really tested and challenged me. It is embarrassing to admit it, but a twelve-minute walk not only wore me out but also left me virtually breathless. One reason I did my walking early in the morning before daylight and by myself was so that no one could see just how out of shape I was! I could barely walk a city block or go up a flight of stairs without getting winded.

I was born with flat feet. Now, when I say *flat feet*, I don't mean just nominally flat; I mean the bone structure in the arches of my feet is essentially inverted. My parents told me regularly that at birth my feet looked so hideously deformed, the doctors first warned them that I might never even walk.

The man who fitted me for my first really good pair of running shoes said my feet were the flattest he'd ever seen in thirty-eight years of business.

These flat feet have bothered me all my life. As a freshman in college, I enrolled in the Reserve Officers' Training Corps (ROTC), but when the ROTC director (an army colonel) saw my feet, he told me there was no point in my continuing because the army wouldn't have me anyway. My flat feet ended what I'm sure would have been a heralded military career in the post-Vietnam 1970s. Frankly, that was just what I needed to hear to further justify my lack of physical activity. I would revel in that for the next thirty years.

My start at running was really accidental. Once I started on my own 12 STOPs experience, I faithfully did several months of only walking, stationary-bike riding, and working out on a weight machine a few days a week. One day, though, I started doing something that I literally had not done since I was in junior high gym class—I started running as well as walking. It was much like the scene from *Forrest Gump* when Forrest was being chased by a group of bullies and, as he started running, his leg braces fell off. I was being chased by a lifetime of bad habits and voices telling me I couldn't, but that day, I found out I *could*! I could never have done that given the condition of my feet except that over the period of nearly a year, my walking had developed strength in me that I previously had not had, and it gave me a new level of stamina that I had never known before. I had no illusions about running marathons or becoming a distance runner. I won't be sprinting my way to a gold medal or winning in the Olympics, but I cannot begin to describe the exhilaration of doing something at the age of forty-eight that I was unable to do even at eighteen!

About a year after I started exercising, I was speaking at a town hall meeting on diabetes with Health and Human Services Secretary Tommy Thompson, and mentioned that I was considering running in a 5K race. A reporter from the Associated Press picked up on it, asked me about it afterward, and put a story on the wire that afternoon headlined, GOVERNOR PLANS ON RUNNING 5K RACE. I was "outed" and then felt I had to do it, but I must confess I was more afraid of that race than I was of running for reelection as governor.

The Firecracker 5K in Little Rock is one of the oldest and

most popular 5Ks in the state. Dr. Kern and my orthopedic surgeon, Dr. Richard Nix (who had done surgery on each of my
knees), recommended it as a good race for beginners because the
terrain is mostly level or slightly downhill, and it's a fun family-
type race. I had never even been to a race, much less run in one,
and was scared senseless that I wouldn't be able to cut it, even
though I was running that distance several times a week. To add
some more pressure, Olympic gold medalist and legendary
marathon runner Joan Benoit Samuelson would be participating
in the race. TV cameras, news photographers, and many ob-
servers would be on board to watch Benoit Samuelson run and
watch me choke! (Or at least, that's the way I figured it.)

The week leading up to the race may have been one of the
most stressful I've ever had. My wife left to help our "baby" girl
of twenty-two—a freshly minted college grad—move to Washington, DC, to begin a job. It was left to me and the dog to get prepared for my first-ever race.

I had no illusions or even crazy thoughts of being competi-
tive. I had a single goal—like Rocky Balboa in the movie, I just
wanted to go the distance.

It rained the morning of the race, and I secretly hoped it
would be called off, but I found out that runners run in the rain.
I arrived early and thought about not getting out of the vehicle,
but my state trooper escort and another trooper who would meet
me at the finish line convinced me that I could not "go wobbly"
now. Lacking any confidence, I lined up near the back so as not
to be run over or laughed at by others. That turned out to be a
mistake—I actually had to slow down because so many ahead of
me were barely moving.

I cannot begin to describe the exhilaration of running that
day! I felt as if I were winning the Super Bowl. When I finished, I

wasn't even out of gas. My spirits were soaring. It was like few moments I'd ever experienced. For most people that day, it was just another race; for me, it was a milestone—an epic, seminal event in my path from fat to fit. Reporters with cameras, notebooks, and microphones crowded around to ask my time. I told them: "It took me forty-eight years, ten months, and nine days to get here!" My actual time was 28:30, 9:14 per mile. Not Olympic, but not bad for a middle-aged guy who could barely walk a year earlier.

A few months after that, I ran another 5K, then an 8K. I improved my per-mile pace to 8:43 in the 8K on a largely uphill course. As I write this book, I'm actually training to run the Little Rock Marathon—26.2 miles! It's amazing to my family and friends, but it's even more amazing to me! It wasn't that I was running against others who paid the entry fee and ran the course. I was racing against *me*—against forty-eight years of bad habits and neglect of my body. Trophies or clocks didn't matter. I was a champion, for I had defeated the most stubborn and challenging foe of all, I overcame *me*!

Maybe you are trying to tell yourself that you will never be able to break the couch-sitting habit and exchange it for an exercise habit. Quit telling yourself that as of *right* now! As someone who spent thirty years lifting little more than a knife and fork and who defined *sit-ups* as scrunching closer to the table for meals and snacks, I can attest to the fact that you can see a dramatic change in the way you approach life, but you have to

STOP SITTING ON THE COUCH.

Dear Governor,

After seeing the many news items regarding your weight loss program and the effects of how much you lost on how you look, it had inspired me to start on a weight loss program of my own. I'm well over 100 pounds of my ideal weight as told to me by my doctor. I also have high blood sugar level considered to be diabetes II. Your promotion of a healthier Arkansas has inspired me to lose the weight I need to and maintain a healthy lifestyle. There is no way I could possibly thank you enough for your commitment to this problem for all Arkansans.

Arkansas

STOP 4

STOP Ignoring Signals from Your Body

The human body is a true marvel. It not only speaks *for* you, but if you listen carefully it speaks *to* you—in fact, it screams to you about how to move toward a new level of personal fitness. In the process, you can regain your health, strength, vigor, and vitality.

As I list some of the signals your body may be sending you, keep in mind that there is a double benefit from heeding these warnings. Not only will it give you revelation and motivation to change bad habits into good ones, but every one of these signals will incrementally disappear as you change the course of your life.

1. **Being tired even when you haven't exerted yourself physically.**

   Fatigue can be caused by a combination of being out of shape and eating foods that cause your blood sugar to jump up and down like a five-foot guard trying to cover Shaquille O'Neal. There is a good chance you attribute being tired to aging–and it's true that as you get older, some capacities do begin to diminish. However, if you are overweight and out of shape, then you are far more tired than you need be.

2. Shortness of breath.
You know you're out of shape when taking a simple flight of stairs or walking from your car to the front door of Wal-Mart causes you to feel as if you've just finished in third place in the Boston Marathon. I used to dread going up the steps at the State Capitol when a gaggle of reporters would be waiting at the top, knowing they would be thrusting microphones in my face and I would be sweating and struggling for enough air to give them answers.

3. Lethargy.
Being tired is one thing, but not really wanting to get up and go can really put a crimp in your job and your life. Fortunately for me, I have enough people pulling me around as if I were on a leash that I rarely have time to react to lethargy. But it's not because I lack the will to wilt! If you are one of those people whose get-up-and-go has gotten up and gone, your body may be trying to tell you something.

4. Depression.
Your body was designed to be active. A sedentary lifestyle is contradictory to the way we are wired and

leads not only to phyiscal atrophy but to emotional and spiritual atrophy as well. Junk food can contribute to depression. But the sense of hopelessness and helplessness from being overweight and out of shape complicates and exaggerates a feeling of worthlessness and creates huge levels of self-doubt. We tend to feel we could never succeed in personal or professional challenges if we can't say no to apple pie! Of course, some people go beyond feeling blue and may experience clinical depression, which needs to be treated by a doctor. Severe depression is the result of chemical imbalances in the brain and cannot be self-treated successfully any more than cancer or heart disease can be. Often well-meaning friends tell a person who is severely depressed to "snap out of it"—which is as ridiculous as telling a person with a broken leg to "just get up and walk and you'll feel better." Whether your depression has gone beyond a mild version—just feeling disappointed and discouraged—to a level needing medical intervention is a question for your doctor to answer. But depression is a clear signal from your body that you shouldn't ignore. I have personally discovered that exercise and good, healthy food are the *best* medicine for mild depression.

5. **Joint and muscle pain.**
   I told my doctor about a pain in my leg and his response was, "It's just old age." That's when I knew I needed to get some additional medical advice—my other leg felt just fine, and it was the same age!

Truth is, many aches and pains are the result not so much of age as of improper maintenance and care of joints and muscles. Since I've started making significant changes in the way I take care of myself, I actually feel significantly younger than when I *was* significantly younger. I'm asked all the time if I find that I have more energy. While the answer to that is yes, it is more than merely the presence of energy. It's the absence of those ever-present nuances of what I had dismissed as "hitting middle age." I'm not kidding myself into thinking that I'm ready to play tackle football or take on a group of high school kids in a pickup basketball game. However, regular exercise keeps the body limber by maintaining the elasticity in the connecting tissue.

Henry Hawk of Conway, Arkansas, is seventy years old and serves on the Governor's Council on Physical Fitness. He recently gave me a calendar he put together. It emphasizes a stretching routine that he has been utilizing for fifty years. He is in superb physical condition, runs in races, and has never had a sports injury after years of running and vigorous exercise. Most thirty-five-year-olds would be happy to trade their strength and agility for those of Henry Hawk. The key to his absence of muscle and joint pain is a faithful, perhaps fanatic commitment to good exercise habits.

6. Restless sleep.

I've never understood why I found it more difficult to get a restful night's sleep when I was tired all the time than I do now after I've worked out and feel great and full of energy at the end of the day. Restless sleep can be one of those signals that your body gives you that shouldn't be ignored. Extremely obese people can experience a condition beyond insomnia and actually suffer from sleep apnea, a common condition in very overweight people that causes your breathing to stop for periods of time. It can be very stressful to the heart and can even be fatal, though it is sometimes mistaken for a heart attack. If your doctor suspects that you are troubled with sleep apnea, he or she may recommend confirming the diagnosis through a sleep clinic and being treated with breathing devices that will work during the night to keep your airway from being disrupted. For overweight people, this kind of sleep disorder is far more than an inconvenience. It can be a deadly medical condition. Even if you don't have a sleep disorder, you will sleep better if you eat right and exercise.

7. **Headaches.**

Loading up on sugary foods and eating an unbalanced diet in general can create headaches and are better cured with a change of lifestyle than a bottle of aspirin. If you're diabetic, your consumption of sugar or of foods that convert to sugar can give you a feeling that your head is a thirty-pounds-per-square-inch tire with fifty pounds of air pumped into it. It's not pleasant, and it's not necessary!

8. **Feeling bloated.**

If you ever felt as if you were going to explode from the inside like an overfilled balloon, you may be experiencing a sense of being bloated. Like the headaches I mentioned before, this is the result of unreleased fluid building up. It can also result in fatigue and light-headedness.

These are just some of the important signals your body may be giving you. It's time to stop ignoring them!

If a close friend who had been a companion for most of your life set you down and gave you loving and helpful advice, it would certainly be rude to completely ignore what the friend was saying. In this case, there is a good chance that your body (which could be your best friend) is trying to give you some very sound advice about the condition you are in and the direction you are headed. Follow the advice you are getting from that trusted friend and

STOP IGNORING SIGNALS FROM YOUR BODY.

DEAR GOVERNOR,

My problem is that I am overweight and need some help. I have watched your progress, and I would love to take off some weight myself. I now weigh 235 and am very depressed about my weight. I grew up in a very abusive home with no support from my parents. I feel I eat when I feel stress! My mom and dad both died from heart attacks and both were overweight. I don't want my children to go through the same pain that I did. I would love to be around them for years to come, and feel healthy doing it.

Thank you,
Arkansas

STOP 5

STOP Listening to Destructive Criticism

If you're overweight, no one has to tap you on the shoulder and let you in on the secret. You know it every time you have to devise a strategy just to tie your shoes. You know it when you put a quarter in one of those fortune-telling scales and, after stepping on, the voice from within says, *One of you guys needs to get off here*! You know it when you get into the car and have to stretch the seat belt to its full extension just to get it around you and you pray that it will actually buckle. You know it from that *swish* sound of your legs rubbing together at the thighs when you walk. You know it because you haven't seen your feet from a standing position in years. (You're pretty sure they're still there because you haven't toppled over.) You know it when you sit in a lawn chair and, upon standing up, have to pull it off you like a tight sock.

But even if you didn't already know that you were out of shape and overweight, there's no need to worry—there are people lined up around the block to tell you about it! Not only will they tell you that you are overweight and need to do something about it, but they will further announce that you *can't* do anything about it and that any attempt you make to change your lifestyle permanently will result in failure. Most of the self-appointed health saviors out there have never struggled with their weight and don't have a clue about an eating obsession.

Listen *very carefully* to what I'm about to tell you because while you *absolutely can change your life patterns*, you can *only* do so if you will heed this very important STOP.

STOP LISTENING TO DESTRUCTIVE CRITICISM.

Chances are, you already have some doubt about your ability to succeed. After all, you have tried before, and you've even tried with some degree of temporary success. You truly worry whether or not you can ever have a breakthrough in your health habits–whether it can become as easy to eat and live healthy as it once was to succumb to every item on the buffet. Truth is, you *can* do it, and for your life to be fun again you *must* do it. But you will have to STOP listening to the "boo birds"–often your closest friends and family members–who have no idea what they are doing to you with their negative and destructive comments.

Some people will probably be unaware of how hurtful their words are because they are in fact simply releasing their own defense mechanisms and reliving their own personal failures. Sad, but true: Some people are more afraid that you will *succeed* than that you will *fail*, for your success presents a threat to them in the area of health or in other parts of their lives where their own choices are out of control. If you are a lifelong foodaholic and are able to change and start along a new course that becomes obvious by your appearance and attitude, it will create a tremendous sense of pressure for others to acknowledge that people *can* change, and that the changes can be permanent and the results can be satisfying. Some of the same people who told me I was fat complained that I had lost too much weight and needed to "put some meat back on my bones." I came to realize that my success in this area of life was like a conviction point to the critic, saying, *Bad behavior can be changed—even yours!*

It has often been said that there is nothing worse than a re-formed anything—a reformed foodaholic, smoker, alcoholic, you name it. Some of your friends will probably dread your success because they fear you will become a "know-it-all" expert and will be judgmental toward them in the same way that others have been judgmental toward you. I've tried to never say to another person who is overweight—"Hey, man, you could use this plan yourself." Unless someone specifically asks me "How did you do it?" I simply graciously acknowledge their kind words about my new appearance and let it go at that.

Almost equal in hurt and discouragement from those who tell you that you *can't* are those who want to tell you how much more successful they've been than you ever will be. You know the type—whatever you have done or accomplished, they are quick to let you know that they have done that, too, but a little bit better. This is the kind of person you pray to God you never sit next to on a long flight overseas or get cornered with at a reception or have to sit near in a doctor's waiting room. Frankly, I would just as soon have gasoline poured down my neck and have what hair I have left set on fire than to endure some boorish person who, upon overhearing that you had a bunion on *your* foot, proceeds to tear off his shoes and socks to show you his!

At all costs, avoid letting yourself being compared with others who have experienced a successful weight loss or lifestyle change! There are many factors that affect how we respond to life changes, not the least of which are our metabolism, our genetic makeup, and the particular plan we are on. Resolve to yourself that your plan is not on anyone's clock or calendar, and that you are willing to be patient because you have determined that you have the rest of your life to get the job done. You may or may not hit a particular artificial weight goal by Christmas or some other self-declared moment, so think long term!

As one who speaks frequently to large and small audiences, I've learned the importance of establishing eye contact with people in the audience who at least outwardly appear to be interested. Admittedly, during some of my speeches, it seems easier to bring peace to the Middle East than to find people who look interested! But looking into the eyes of those who are smiling, are nodding (hopefully not nodding off to sleep), and have that look of focus is critical to being able to deliver a decent speech. I call these audience members my "anchors" because even though I may try to look around the room and make eye contact with everyone, I will go again and again to those faces of calm and reassurance who keep me encouraged, confident, and focused. Find some "anchors" who believe in you and will encourage you. These may *not* be family members or close friends. Don't assume you'll get the best support from those closest to you. A support group like the one offered by Weight Watchers (or the UAMS program I followed) may be your best bet because it will formalize those anchors.

Earlier I told you to be sure to set a start date, share that date with others, and then start your plan. Those with whom you share your commitment who are positive and encouraging could be considered your anchors. Make sure you keep regular contact with them even if it's informal and even if it has nothing to do with your health regimen. You will want to hear from them simple words of encouragement–anything from "Hey, you've lost some weight, you're looking good," to simple inquiries like "How's it going? Are you hanging in there?"

What you *don't* want to do is to hang around those people who will say, "Yeah, my uncle tried to lose weight and after three weeks he dropped dead of a heart attack. His whole family said he would have been better off just eating what he wanted."

Hopefully your immediate family will encourage you, but don't count on it! Perhaps if you've tried and failed before, they have little confidence that this time will be any different. They may actually resent that your lifestyle changes will affect what's for dinner, where you take them out to eat, and whether or not you stop for pie on the way home from the movies. If other members of your family are also struggling, your efforts and–even more so–your success will only cause them to confront their own needs for healthy behavior. And they may not want to deal with it.

As important as it is to not listen to destructive criticism, it's equally vital that you avoid the self-righteous attitudes and conversations of those around you. Avoid ever telling people what they should do or telling them they should join you in your efforts.

Many people will say, "Boy, I need to lose some weight myself." They are not looking for you to say, "You sure do. If there ever was a person who looks like she could sink a ship by standing on the end of it–it would be you!" No, this person is probably just trying to be nice; the only response you need to give is "Thank you very much. I know it was quite a challenge for me." That way, you are not telling her that she looks great when she doesn't; nor are you being judgmental and telling her she's a fat blob. But you are acknowledging that whatever she feels is beyond your capacity to evaluate. You simply are aware of what *you* had to do.

You will have other well-meaning friends who believe they are encouraging you when they tell you that you can do it only if you use whatever plan they used. If they succeeded with the Atkins diet, they will swear it's the only way in the world to lose weight. If they've gone on the American Diabetes Association diet, they will announce *it* is the only safe and healthy way. If they've enrolled in a Weight Watchers course, they might say that while other methods can work, Weight Watchers is by far the best.

As I've said earlier and want to say again—be less concerned about the *vehicle* you use than you are about the *destination.* Your focus should not be on losing weight but on getting healthy. While there are some basic principles of diet and nutrition that will help you to be successful over the long haul, it has as much to do with what you feed your mind as it does with what you feed your body! If you feed your mind the right food of encouragement and factual information, you will find it much easier to feed your body the healthy foods that actually cause you to lose weight, feel better, and regain your health.

Many successful programs include support group meetings. My schedule and situation made weekly meetings impractical, but I had "electronic meetings" with my doctor, nutritionist, and trusted friends via e-mail. Accountability is critical! Knowing someone is going to ask me how I'm doing forces me to do better.

You won't have to look very hard to find people who discourage you, disappoint you, or depress you. But when you find those who help you by their kind words and positive reinforcement, keep in contact with them. Faithfully follow this important STOP along the way to forever fitness:

STOP LISTENING TO DESTRUCTIVE CRITICISM.

DEAR GOVERNOR,

I saw you on the CBS Early Show interview about your weight loss and changes in lifestyle. I felt inspired to let you know that I was moved by your achievements. I weighed 372 lbs. at my highest point and have shed 32 lbs. in a little over three months. I continue to work hard at my weight loss, and when I feel I'm at a plateau, I look at your interview again and again. While Gov. Arnold [Schwarzenegger] has always been in great shape I feel I cannot relate to him. You, however, I can relate to and I find your story very inspirational. Please keep up the good work and healthy lifestyle. Thank you for sharing your story.

California

STOP 6

STOP Expecting Immediate Success

M*any aspire, few attain.* This sums up the experiences of many who have squared their feet in the starting blocks but never known the joy of breaking the tape at the finish line. My hope and prayer is that you will experience the finish line and not just another well-intentioned beginning that concludes in failure, frustration, and additional fat.

From my own experience, a common problem is expecting immediate success. This kind of thinking can actually work against you rather than for you in the long run.

Rapid weight loss often occurs in the early days of a health plan: It's not uncommon to lose a fairly significant amount of weight in the first ten days. Depending on your age and other factors, such as personal metabolism and total body mass index, you might lose as much as seven to ten pounds in the first week. While doctors may be dismissive of such an initial spurt by calling it "water loss," it sure looks good on the scale—and it may give you a false hope that if seven pounds can be shed in the first week, you should be able to lose twenty-eight pounds or more in a month! While that may in fact happen for some on a very strict and radical diet, there's a greater likelihood that weight loss will come in waves.

After dramatic initial success, you may actually go a week or more following a very strict regimen and not lose any weight. Then the next week you'll suddenly drop four or five pounds. It is also possible for your weight to fluctuate as much as five pounds a day, which can be attributed to water retention or other factors that your doctor can explain far better than I could.

Frankly, *weight loss* can often be acquired rather quickly, but *health* will take a while. Remember, your goal is not next month's reunion, but added years and a better quality of life. There's a good chance that you've spent years developing the unhealthy habits that led to an unhealthy body. The process of change can begin within minutes and hours from the time you decide. Some results can be seen within days or weeks. But don't let anyone kid you into thinking you can give yourself twelve weeks to completely change all your habits, then, at the end of this period, put your feet up, relax, and consider your job complete!

If you wear glasses, for instance, chances are that you're going to need some type of assistance in correcting your vision for the rest of your life. Even if you get rid of your glasses and switch to contact lenses or have the latest eye surgery, you're still confronting some kind of deterioration of your vision. If you wear dentures, your teeth will not grow back—the dentures are for life. If you have a hearing aid, unless some surgery either exists or is developed that completely restores your hearing, that hearing aid will be a part of you for as long as you live and wish to hear what others are saying.

Don't be depressed or discouraged when I tell you that your goal is not merely the loss of a prescribed number of pounds. I've been through many attempts at weight loss in the past, but one fundamental difference I experienced when I enrolled in the program at UAMS was that I was determined to regain my health and did not set a specific target for weight loss. While I realize this may seem totally contradictory to most weight loss approaches, I also knew there are inherent dangers in targeting a certain amount of weight as if it's the secret to good health. There is no question excess weight is unhealthy, but it isn't the only indicator of poor health. In fact, many experts on the aging process note that it's better to be "fat and fit" than it is to be thin and terribly out of shape.

One of the world's leading experts on aging is Dr. David A. Lipschitz, professor of geriatrics at the University of Arkansas for Medical Sciences and director of the Donald W. Reynolds Center on Aging in Little Rock. He hosts the popular series on PBS called *Aging Successfully with Dr. David* and is a breakthrough visionary on the effects and issues of aging. The first chapter of *Breaking the Rules of Aging*, his delightful and entertaining book, is actually titled "Don't Lose Weight!"

Now, before you gleefully go out and purchase his book and expect Dr. Lipschitz to tell you that you can keep all those unneeded and unnecessary pounds, please understand the real message: Fitness involves a great deal more than just what's revealed on the bathroom scales. There are some overweight people who are much healthier than some of their rail-thin friends.

My goal throughout this process has been to become a healthy and fit person, not to reach someone else's definition of an ideal weight. Throughout my pilgrimage, people would ask, "How much weight do you plan to lose?" To which I always replied, "I'm not sure—wherever my body takes me once I have achieved a level of health."

News reporters in Arkansas have followed my dramatic change of behavior and appearance very carefully. After all, it's difficult to hide the loss of more than a hundred pounds when you're photographed hundreds of times each day and your picture is on television and in the newspapers on a daily basis.

One reporter who took a keen interest in my progress was Caryn Rousseau of the Associated Press. She had requested an opportunity to interview me while I was approaching the milestone of fifty pounds of weight loss. She actually came along with an AP photographer to the Governor's Mansion at four thirty one morning to walk with me around the track and talk with me about what I was doing and why. As it turned out, Caryn had experienced a dramatic transformation in her own life years earlier. She had lost some sixty pounds since graduating from high school in Indiana. She is a very petite and attractive young lady, and I couldn't imagine her weighing much more than a hundred pounds total. But I knew that she, unlike most, would actually understand what I was going through. In fact, she became a tremendous source of encouragement and inspiration to me. I wished I had made the changes in my life in my twenties instead of my late forties. Caryn now runs several miles daily, participates in races and marathons, and is the picture of health, having maintained it for several years. Her follow-up stories have made the national wire, and in 2004 her stories on my weight loss and regained health won her press awards. Of all the reporters who've asked me about my weight loss, Caryn was the only one who understood why I never announced a weight goal: From her own experience, she had already learned what I was learning–that the issue is not so much weight but health and fitness.

Just as the alcoholic must give up alcohol and consider sobriety a *lifetime* decision, so the foodaholic must give up the habits of unhealthy eating and behavior and make it a lifetime effort. One major difference, of course, is that a person can live without alcohol–and hopefully was not introduced to it as an infant!–but food is a necessity. We started eating before we can remember, and we cannot simply quit. We have to learn how to change our eating habits and develop new types of craving. The really good news is that just as our body learned how to crave junk food and developed an insatiable appetite for unhealthy things, that same body can be *retrained* and in the process our health *regained*.

While you will certainly want to keep up with your weight changes, try to avoid the temptation of weighing yourself every single day, because if you go three or four days with very strict food consumption and exercise, and then don't experience a single ounce of weight loss (in fact, you may experience a pound or two of gain), you may be tempted to say, "This new approach isn't working. I might as well eat a half gallon of ice cream tonight!"

In addition to the speedometer, there are many different gauges on the dashboard of your car that you need to keep your eye on to know what kind of shape your car is in. If you don't look at the gas gauge, oil indicator, oil pressure, and other important indicators, you might find yourself stranded on the side of the road. When it comes to your body, there are also several "gauges" you need to keep your eye on. Earlier I suggested that you go to your doctor to get a good medical checkup and analysis so you will have a baseline with which to compare your progress. Blood pressure, blood sugar, cholesterol level, A1C hemoglobin index, and heart rate are all factors you need to focus on more than just weight. Even so, over time you will very likely reverse dangerous trends if you truly follow a pattern of good behavior regarding what you eat and how you exercise. But it's best that you consider these observations and check them once a month rather than once a day.

An old expression—*up like a rocket and down like a rock*—describes many people who've experienced rapid weight loss but also seen a subsequent rapid weight gain. This type of yo-yo dieting (which I have experienced in the past) is dangerous to your health and usually results in a weight gain that exceeds the previous high. This is also very discouraging and leads to a sense of despair and hopelessness about ever being healthy.

It takes about nine months from conception until the birth of a baby. Most college degrees require at least four years of study. It takes months of careful attention to simply grow some vegetables in a backyard garden. Don't be fooled into thinking that a lifetime of unhealthy behavior will change into a lifestyle of healthy behavior in a few days, weeks, or even months. Take the pressure off yourself to achieve someone else's image of you. Expect that over the next several months or even years, you will lose weight, you will look healthy, you will be able to shop in the regular section instead of the big-and-tall section. But gauge your success not so much by the numbers that will show up on your scale as by the sense of satisfaction and self-worth you attain from having changed your habits and the direction of your health. That's why it's important to nail down this STOP on your way to "forever fitness":

STOP EXPECTING IMMEDIATE SUCCESS.

DEAR GOVERNOR,

I loved what you said about having to look at food differently and to stop blaming others. I think people need to be accountable for themselves, and I believe that people can be more aware of health. In the summer of 2002, my husband at age 33 had severe chest pain and I rushed him to the hospital. Luckily it was not heart trouble, but it was a big wake-up call for him. He was over 300 lbs. and that was probably the cause of some pain along with the heat of the day and other things. So he was determined to lose weight and become fit. After a year, he had lost 100 lbs. and continues to lose weight and tone up. The biggest thing he added to his get-fit routine was exercise—walking and riding a bike.

With your wake-up call, you have begun to help the people of Arkansas with "Healthy Arkansas" and make a difference in many lives.

Kentucky

STOP 7

STOP Whining

Sydney Case is a delightful, remarkably upbeat person whom I appointed to serve on the Governor's Council on People with Disabilities. She has been a tremendous member of that commission, providing positive leadership to the issues facing those with disabilities. Because her attitude and outlook are contagious, she infects all those around her with a sense of joy and optimism. Sydney has been confined to a wheelchair for many years. But her body is the only thing that is confined about this marvelous lady.

One day during an event at the Governor's Mansion where Sydney was present, I happened to notice a sticker attached to the back of her wheelchair. It got my attention and touched my heart because in bold letters it simply read NO WHINING! Through the process of learning how to retrain my mind and body for healthy habits, I thought often of Sydney and her trademark expression. It has helped me, and I believe it will help you.

Through the years, I've often given motivational speeches

and encouraged people to think positively. Studies have confirmed what many individuals have known from their own experiences—a positive attitude has healing properties.

One of the most powerful medicines we will ever take is derived from the simple act of laughing. Laughter is a sign of a positive mind-set. You don't genuinely laugh when you're miserable. Furthermore, the physical act of laughing actually releases endorphins into your adrenal system, helping to alleviate pain and triggering a sense of alertness.

I often use humor in speeches, not only to gain an audience's attention but also to help them relax, listen more carefully, and remember the message I'm trying to convey. It works. People come up to me and remind me of a story I told in a speech years ago. (Frankly, I don't even remember the event! But they remember the *story*.)

As you begin major changes in your lifestyle, there will be strong temptations to look at a menu and lament all those things you *cannot* have. You might eye a buffet of delicious food and gaze longingly at those items packed with calories that you know are off limits, and feel a sense of deprivation and loss. Learning to change your attitude toward food, health, exercise, and lifestyle is critical to long-term success, and it can't be accomplished if you don't STOP WHINING.

Let's face it—no one wants to be around a chronic whiner. There are some people who can find the negative in anything and everything. Most of us would rather place a pair of diaperless twin babies in our laps an hour after lunch than have to endure much time around a person who believes every day with sunshine is a day to get sunburned, and every day with rain is just a day to get wet.

Attitude determines our altitude. People who are convinced they can't accomplish something will find their attitude to be a self-fulfilling prophecy. I am not suggesting you artificially act pleasant in the face of tragedy or genuine disappointment. But adopting the can-do spirit, surrounding yourself with positive reinforcement and encouraging friends is essential to success.

Don't talk yourself into believing that you're some kind of martyr for making these lifestyle changes. You will probably feel tempted to make a list of things you can't eat or can't do anymore. I would suggest that this is a huge mistake! Instead, make a list of the foods you *can* eat and the things you *can* and in fact *must* do. Many of my friends have asked if it was difficult for me to quit eating desserts, candies, and large portions of fatty fried foods and junk foods. I found myself honestly saying that I have not felt deprived. The reason is that I determined early on that my deprivation would not be foods that I once craved. Instead, I would deprive myself of an early heart attack, or having toes or feet amputated because of diabetes. I would deprive myself of completely avoidable disabilities such as loss of sight, stroke, or even premature death by making positive changes in my behavior.

I never thought I would be able to say this, but the truth is, I would now rather have an apple than a candy bar. I have trained my tastes so that the candy bar is not even a serious temptation anymore. There is no way I can convey to you what a radical reversal of attitudes this is—and *you can reverse these attitudes, too!*

At the risk of sounding as repetitive as a scene from Bill Murray's movie *Groundhog Day,* if you don't already have one, you need a definite and positive support group as you begin the process of retooling your appetite. Whether you engage in a more formalized structure like Weight Watchers or a model similar to the program I was a part of at the University of Arkansas for Medical Sciences, you most certainly need to have regular, chronic, and consistent contact with people who will help you "STOP whining about your dining" and give you the encouragement to burn new patterns into your mind that will become instinct and routine.

Throughout this book, I have mentioned some specific things that I have either done myself or known others to do. I've tried to steer clear of an absolute prescriptive model because that is exactly why many (including me) have failed in previous attempts to change health habits. We tend to focus on the "machinery of our method" rather than on changing our minds and therefore refocusing our motivation. Before we change our behavior, we have to change our thinking. A critical part of changing our thinking is believing what we are doing is far better than the life we were living before.

The word *repentance* is familiar to people who have been brought up in or regularly attend church. It essentially means a person makes a 180-degree turn, repenting from a life of "sinful behavior" to a life of "righteous behavior." You might say that a successful change of health habits is true repentance.

Billy Sunday, the famous and flamboyant evangelist of the last century, was known for his powerful sermons and clever rejoinders to critics. One day, a lady offended by the bluntness of one of his sermons stomped up toward him and declared, "Mr. Sunday, I do not like what you are preaching. You've rubbed the cat's fur the wrong way!" Billy Sunday simply replied, "Then, lady, turn the cat around!"

What we have to learn to do is to STOP feeling that diet and exercise are loathsome tortures brought about by our being bad people and instead start realizing that our positive change of behavior is proof that we have strength to do *anything*; that in fact, we are empowered to take charge of our bodies and make them work *for* us rather than work *against* us. You're worth changing! Believe that your life is too valuable to break down, so you're giving it the attention you deserve!

If someone offers you dessert when you have chosen not to eat, don't say, "Oh, I can't have that." Learn to say, "That looks delicious, but I'd rather pass it up because everything else I've eaten today is so very good and I'm full." When someone says, "Would you like some bread?" don't reply, "No, I can't have that bread." Instead, say, "The bread looks and smells absolutely wonderful, but there are so many good things to enjoy, I just can't get to all of it. Thank you, though." Always look for a way to make a positive response even when you have to say no. It will help train your mind to cooperate with your body. *Accept the fact that you are not working toward depriving yourself and missing something, but instead working toward delighting yourself and gaining something—longer life, better appearance, and your health.*

If you have gotten this far, then hopefully you believe more and more that this is a realistic and reachable goal—and it is. But like the other STOPs along the way, don't forget to

STOP WHINING.

DEAR GOVERNOR,

Thank you for sharing your inspiring story in the August 2004 issue of People *magazine. I have just begun my personal journey of weight loss this week. Your story gives me so much hope and enthusiasm. I will remove it from the magazine and save it among my favorite weight loss inspiration stories that I know I will need for inspiration when I hit the low days in my health program. Thank you again, Governor Huckabee.*

Florida

STOP 8

STOP Making Exceptions

Are you doomed never to taste ice cream again? Will eating a chocolate bar cause you to get the shakes? Will a big bowl of biscuits and gravy cause your body to convulse? Of course not! Still, while you may choose to occasionally indulge in "forbidden foods" sometime in the future, during this period of retraining your body and mind it is quite important that you STOP making exceptions.

Even after a few days and certainly a few weeks on a very strict regimen of behavior changes, you will be tempted to cheat—even if only a little bit. Don't do it! The road to ruin is a short one, and it begins by making the mistake early in your program of deciding that you can go off the course "just a little" and easily get back on the road. Instead, visualize that the road you are on has steep shoulders on either side; for the next several miles of travel, getting off that road could well lead to a loss of control and a major wreck. Will there ever be a time in your future when you will enjoy an occasional diversion and dive headfirst into a cheeseburger? Probably so, but it's far better to make sure you don't anytime soon. I would suggest that you are not ready to have it until you reach the place where you don't feel you really need it.

After I'd gone for a full year without eating a single cheeseburger, I realized if I really wanted one, I could have it. But the difference was *I really didn't want it.* After that period of time, I could have taken a bite of one and not suddenly felt I was about to go into a food binge and be forced to keep eating it until I finished off the last crumb. But I honestly didn't want one!

It is important for you to prove to yourself that you really will not die by skipping dessert. Instead of asking yourself whether you can make an exception, create a game of specifically and deliberately declining things just to prove to yourself that you can. If you know you are going to attend a wedding reception where there will be a long table of absolutely irresistible food, tell yourself before you go that no matter what, no matter how many times your Aunt Edna approaches you with a plateful of food, you'll decline. Even if she begs you to try it because she made it just for you, know that under no circumstances will you touch a single bit of food. Even if there are things on the table that you could very safely eat, your purpose is to realize that you don't need to eat any of it in order to feel satisfied.

In the initial stages of my habit breaking, I attended many events. No matter how many times or ways I was offered food, even perfectly healthy options, I simply declined so I could get into the habit of saying, "No thank you." Previously when I had gone to similar events and indulged myself in virtually everything on the table, I left having enjoyed the food but feeling terribly guilty for overeating. Now I experience a complete opposite pleasure: the ability to "go but say no." The exhilaration from having successfully declined the food was far more thrilling than any food I have ever eaten! The feeling of empowerment that comes from actually having control over your appetite is its own most powerful reward.

Let me emphasize that this is training–repeating actions over and over until your actions are "reactions" that are predictable. That marks a new habit!

I was even able to get through the long holiday period between Thanksgiving and the Super Bowl I mentioned earlier. Every day that I was able to resist the temptation before me was a day in which I grew stronger and felt better. It became easier and easier to make my choices by instinct and natural reactions. Even if you are with a group of people who are all grabbing for doughnuts, you will feel ten feet tall when you resist the temptation and say no to what others are saying yes to.

Until you reach the point where temptations have no effect on you, I suggest you make no exceptions–no matter what. It may not, however, be realistic to avoid every temptation every day. Especially if your grandmother stayed up all night making your favorite coconut pie and insists that you not break her heart by refusing it. If you find yourself in such a situation, eat only a few bites and gain the satisfaction of knowing what you were willing to say no to.

Should you find yourself in a very tough predicament where you anticipate it will be difficult to say no and keep from offending your host, then make plans for the dietary detour at least a week in advance. Anticipate that you will indeed fall off the wagon for a specified period of time and for a very specific reason and then immediately upon concluding the exception go right back to a very strict routine.

It is very important not to make an exception on impulse no

matter what the occasion may be. It's true some people are very pushy when it comes to food and can't seem to take no for an answer. If you don't feel you can simply say to someone, "I wouldn't care for any," you can always blame it on your medical condition or your doctor: "That looks delicious and I would love to have some, but my doctor has made me promise I would not have any sugar until at least after my next checkup." Or you can say, "I'm taking something. I'll have to indulge another time." (You're *taking* control of your eating, so you aren't lying, but it gets you off the hook.)

When Harry Smith of CBS's *Early Show* interviewed me, he asked me if I ever cheated. I tried to explain that I didn't cheat—and occasionally going "off program" is not "cheating."

If you study the physiological reaction your body has to foods with a high glycemic index such as potatoes, breads, pastas, or processed foods, you will realize why it's so hard to say no. Once you start eating those foods, it's easy to feel compelled to continue eating until you simply cannot hold any more. One of the main reasons why you should avoid the exceptions is that a food with a high glycemic index triggers a spike in blood sugar and makes it more and more difficult to say no. It almost creates a druglike addiction—a compulsion to eat more of the very foods your body should be saying no to. Just as alcoholics must rid themselves of alcohol by going through a detox period, you also need to give your body time to adjust. In the first few weeks of an effective change of diet, you need to truly detox your body from the foods, additives, and chemicals it is used to craving and instead retrain it with healthy whole foods. You will find that many of your tastes will change dramatically over time.

All this is not to say that in the early days, you should try to eat things that you hate. Eating should and will be a real pleasure and an activity from which you will receive much enjoyment. As your body goes through physiological changes and begins to adjust your desires to different choices, it becomes exceptionally important not to bend or yield to the foods you have been devouring most of your life. In the first three months of my intense weight loss phase, I utilized meal replacements mostly in the form of shakes or soups and limited solid foods to salads and vegetables. It helped me break my poor eating habits.

Don't betray yourself by deciding that since you are going be eating in restaurants, you will be forced to make exceptions. It might require some creativity and resourcefulness on your part, but you will do whatever you choose to do.

I doubt you travel as much as I do or are faced with as many meals you have no control over as I am. I have a regular routine that requires me to speak at breakfast, lunch, and dinner meetings. Even if the items put before me are not things I can eat, I can generally request something from the kitchen staff, and they are usually most happy to help. I confess that being a governor sometimes creates some special treatment. Larry, the food service manager at the fabulous Peabody Hotel in Little Rock, knows I hate carrots. No matter the occasion at the Peabody or adjacent Statehouse Convention Center—where I attend something every week at least—Larry sees to it that if twelve hundred plates are served with carrots, my plate has an alternative! You might have to work a bit if you don't have a helper who's as much a perfectionist as my friend Larry, but you can do it.

Another option is to request a vegetarian plate. If the vegetables are prepared by steaming or grilling, this almost always provides a healthy and delicious alternative. While I'm too much of a carnivore to want to do this very often, it points up that you can take control of what you eat, even when eating out or traveling.

I realize that this becomes somewhat more challenging while engaging in business lunches or dinners because you may not get to select the place or even the menu. Still, it's a cop-out to say you are "forced" to eat unhealthy things, because you are most certainly not. If all else fails, order a small dinner salad without dressing and take your time eating small bites of it. I've heard the excuse, "I didn't want to offend my host or client so I ate everything the waiter brought." Nonsense! The ultimate offense is not taking care of yourself. Learn to cheerfully eat what you need and only what you should and you'll not offend others.

I have often requested salads with certain ingredients left off. I quit using salad dressing, opting either for simple seasoning like salt, pepper, and other spices or perhaps salsa as a substitute for salad dressing. I used to believe that a salad had as its primary purpose adding some bulk to a bowl of buttermilk ranch dressing. I now love salad without globs of dressing that cover up the taste of the vegetables and wonder why I didn't eat it that way all the years before. It's no longer a matter of feeling I'm on some special diet that causes me to say no to certain foods. I have methodically detoxed my body from the cravings of the past and retrained it to actually want the things that are healthy, and to be completely satisfied by them.

If you do mess up and fall to a temptation, don't despair, and for sure don't convince yourself that you are incapable of success and might as well go ahead and go full-speed back to the old habits! If you acted on an impulse, admit to yourself and to others around you that it was a mistake. Decide it really wasn't that good and certainly not worth that feeling of failure and guilt you have experienced. Tell yourself that you will not only avoid that mistake again but also learn from it and not allow yourself to be placed at the same point of temptation again. It is very helpful to ask a friend or family member to call your attention to your behavior should you begin acting as if you are going to ignore the commitment you have made. There is a tremendous sense of accomplishment when one day you realize that you intuitively look at the salads on the menu without even paying attention to the desserts, which may be the polar opposite of your former habits.

I hope you are beginning to gain confidence in your capacity to be healthy and live with the strength and vitality you may not have known since you were a child. But I also know that in order to get there, you need to heed carefully this STOP along the way and

STOP MAKING EXCEPTIONS.

Dear Governor,

I just want to thank you for your weight loss program. I, too, am 48 years old and was 110 [pounds] overweight. In January I had two of my doctors tell me that I must lose the weight as I was on the verge of having some major medical problems. However, I still could not get motivated. I had several friends who had never had weight problems die unexpectedly this spring, so basically my attitude was "What the heck, I'm going to die anyway, I might as well eat what I like." I was depressed. Then I saw an article about the weight loss program you were on. It was the inspiration that I needed to make the first stop. I started a program about 10 weeks ago and am now glad to say I've lost 48 lbs. I know I still have a long way to go, but I know I can do it. I have had the support of family, friends, and co-workers, and the inspiration provided by you.

Mississippi

STOP 9

STOP Storing Provisions for Failure

One reason so many of us fail in our attempt to lose weight is that we do more to plan for failure than we do to plan for success. You will ultimately accomplish what you prepare for. As you prepare for success, you will succeed. But if you plan for failure—even if it's not a conscious decision to do so—you will inevitably fail. You may wonder why. In this chapter, we are going to explore one of the simple secrets that will keep us from failing.

My dad was a fireman in Hope, Arkansas, and we lived in a small rented house just two blocks from the fire station. I spent a great deal of my childhood hanging around the fire station talking to firemen, sliding down the pole, ringing the bell on the fire engines, and listening to firemen talk about fires, how they started, and how to put them out.

A fire must have two essential ingredients in order to burn. It must have fuel–whether that be wood, fabric, gasoline, or synthetic material–and it must have air. When a fire is deprived of either of these two essentials, it goes out. Likewise, in order to continue your out-of-shape, overweight, and out-of-control condition, two ingredients are crucial. One is your *appetite*, and the other is giving yourself *access* to the kind of fuel that will increase your appetite while adding little or no nutritional value and storing calories in the form of fat. It really isn't necessary for you to starve yourself in order to lose weight. In fact, as I was taught the fundamentals of nutrition, I made the amazing discovery that one of the worst strategies you can practice is skipping meals. I know many people who believe if they cut one or two meals a day they will lose weight, then are shocked when they either remain static or, worse, actually gain weight while eating less.

If you already have a strong appetite (and most likely you do or you wouldn't be reading this book and battling the bulge!), there is a good chance your appetite has increased not only because of how much you eat, but also due to the specific *kinds* of things you eat. Foods that have a high glycemic index cause your blood sugar to spike and then rapidly crash, leaving you wanting more and creating an insatiable appetite even if your body does not need any additional calories for fuel. If you can get your appetite under control, you are well on your way to a changed lifestyle. But that is very unlikely to happen unless you confront the second major "fat essential": *access* to high-calorie, high-glycemic-index, and low-nutrition foods.

Have you ever kept a diary of what you eat on any given day? If you actually recorded everything you ate, you would be surprised how many times you reached for the unplanned, unexpected snack or went into the refrigerator for "just a bite of something."

One of the hardest habits for me to break was that of STOR-ING PROVISIONS FOR FAILURE.

Let me be blunt: If you can stop storing provisions for failure, you will have made a quantum leap toward permanent lifestyle changes, and it will further assist not only curbing your appetite but completely reshaping it so you will be craving an apple or some strawberries instead of a bowl of ice cream or a bag of potato chips! Sound impossible? I thought so, too. But of all the miracles I have experienced, none has surprised me more than finding out that restricting *access* and controlling *appetite* are true secrets to permanent behavior change.

Without lying to yourself or cheating, start looking around to see how many different food items you have stashed in a variety of places. My guess is that your desk drawer at work (or your locker at school if you are a student) is but one of the many places where you keep candy, gum, chips, or even change in the specific amount needed for a nearby vending machine. Take a good look at what's inside your refrigerator and freezer and the cabinets in your kitchen. The fact that there are unhealthy foods present may not be as revealing as will be your awareness of it and your regular if not at least occasional venture toward it to stave off a craving. Even in your car, there's probably a place where you keep a few snacks stored just for those occasions when nothing is open and you need something to eat (or at least so you have told yourself). Now I'm going to suggest you do something that you will find very hard to do, and my guess is you won't do it at first. Still, I urge you to rethink the idea and do exactly as I recommend: Get rid of the food that you have stashed and by so doing STOP storing provisions for failure.

I can almost guarantee that if you keep these foods on hand

(even though you have told yourself you can't have them any-more), it won't be weeks or months but only days from now when after a harsh comment from a colleague or family member, you will find refuge in them.

It may be the moment in which you find your weight has gone up instead of down for the second consecutive day despite your best attempts to eat right. Or it could be the day you received especially distressing news. No matter; you will do what has been your habit to do all those many years when confronted with a crisis. You have always found comfort by eating—but not just any kind of eating. You found comfort in eating foods so lacking in nutritional value that you would probably be better off eating the package and throwing away the food. These foods are so familiar that they have felt almost like your "friend." In a stressful moment, you feel as if an angel sits on one shoulder saying "no" and a demon sits on the other saying "yes."

In a split second of impulse, you are ripping open the wrapper and devouring hundreds of calories you neither planned nor need. And what's worse is that this will not be the only thing you tear into once you start. You might consume a second and third consecutive snack in a matter of minutes, and after that it only gets easier. By this time you've convinced yourself if you're going to "blow it," you might as well go all the way. You continue eating until either you have exhausted your stored provisions or you are so completely overwhelmed with calories (albeit unhealthy and empty ones) that you are on the brink of being physically ill. Not only do you now find yourself not wanting to even waddle across the room, but you've also added to your sense of guilt by completely violating the pledge you made to yourself. Now you're second-guessing how on earth you could have gotten so out of control, gotten there so quickly, and stayed there so completely.

If necessary, you may try replacing your stash of empty calories with nutritious snacks such as fruit cups without syrup, plain nuts, or even carrot or celery sticks with no-fat ranch dressing in the refrigerator.

There is a biological truth you must confront. Once you started eating those calories, it sent your blood sugar soaring like an F-16 on maneuvers. The only thing that was likely to stop it was when you finally ran out of fuel. Had you not stored those provisions for failure, you might not have succumbed to the first bite and could have avoided not only a disastrous crash in your plan but all the guilt that goes with it as well.

Maybe you can't bring yourself to throw away the candy, the chips, and all the other junk food because drilled into your mind are all your parents' admonitions about "all the hungry children of the world." If so, then give this food away to your skinny friends or those who have not yet made such a commitment, but *at all cost and however you must do it, get that food completely away from you!*

Remember that the kinds of foods you eat can dramatically speed up or slow down your *appetite*, and your *access* to those foods will in all probability dictate whether you stand or fall. One dirty little secret is that you are not as likely to engage in a "pig-out" in front of friends, family, or co-workers if they know you're trying to change your habits. You are not at your greatest risk dining out with friends at a nice restaurant or attending a reception where there are numerous buffet tables loaded with off-limits foods. You are *most* vulnerable when you are all by yourself and when you think no one is watching or will ever know. But then maybe you've forgotten that *you* will know, and all the food you just consumed did not equal in good taste how bad you feel physically and emotionally.

So although it may seem like a small thing, it is critical that you

STOP STORING PROVISIONS FOR FAILURE.

DEAR GOVERNOR,

I just saw on nationwide TV news about your courageous recovery from obesity. What an inspiration you are for all of us! Congratulations to you! Leadership takes form in many shapes; you have shown true leadership to your fortunate constituents as well as folks like me in far-off Washington State. My very best to you and my most sincere thanks for your truly inspirational leadership.

Washington State

STOP 10

STOP Fueling with Contaminated Food

In an earlier chapter, I confessed that one of my personal pleasures is my passion for bass fishing–made all the more pleasant by the ownership of a bass boat. For the uninitiated, the twenty-one-foot Bass Cat Jaguar that I have is a high-performance boat that sits low in the water and is designed for getting you to a particular fishing hole at speeds comparable to those achieved on a NASCAR track. My boat is powered by a 225-horsepower Mercury OptiMax outboard. I have achieved speeds well over eighty miles an hour, and because of the nature of the engine, I have to use premium-quality gasoline with an octane rating of ninety-two or above. I'm very particular about what goes into that engine because I know I can't afford to replace it, and I know that its ability to run at optimum performance is directly linked to the quality of fuel that it is fed. I wouldn't pour dirty water, soda, or even cheap gas in that engine.

Why should I take care of a boat and abuse my body?

It should not come as a big surprise that in order to achieve a level of health and fitness and therefore maintain this incredible engine called the human body, the type of fuel we give ourselves is of immense importance. It determines to a large degree how well our bodies perform and how long they will last.

I doubt that you'd ever take a seat in a busy restaurant and suggest to the waitress that she not bring additional plates, cups, or utensils, because you'll just use those that are already on the table from the previous diners. The very thought is disgusting— even if the people eating before you were your own family. (For some of you, *especially* if they were your own family!) We insist on clean plates, forks, knives, spoons, and cups, and we should. We don't want the unnecessary contamination of someone else's germs.

Even though dogs are known to drink from the toilet bowl, I personally don't know anyone, no matter how thirsty he or she may be, who has done so. In fact, my dog, a wonderful black Lab named Jet, is so particular that he will not drink from the toilet bowl, either. (I'm especially grateful for this during those moments when he jumps up on me and gives me one of those Labrador-retriever-size licks across the face.)

We take good care of our boats and cars, and even insist that the water we run through our washing machine or dishwasher is clean and pure.

Maybe you own a car that you love and treat like your child. It doesn't make a great deal of sense, but the fact is, we're often more particular about vehicles that we expect to replace every four or five years than we are with our bodies, which can't be replaced!

If you can participate in a food plan that very thoroughly lists each day exactly what you are to eat and to the ounce how much, then congratulations and *bon appétit.* I will confess that one reason I found such a food plan difficult was that I'm not someone who'll measure the weight or count the calories of everything I eat. I never feel I have the time—and sometimes I can simply be too stubborn to be that rigid. Now, if it works for you, then you should for sure do it, and I admire those for whom this comes easy. For me, it's much easier to create an overall list of things I can't eat and the things I should, and then choose only from the list of can-do food. As for portions, I go by the simple rule that if it's larger than my fist, it's too large.

Let me list some things that probably should be on your own "contaminated fuel list."

1. **Refined sugar.**

   To be blunt, your body doesn't need it, and you need to eliminate it. You will not die from a lack of it, but you most certainly could die from an abundance of it. If there are certain sweet things you feel you must have, several good sugar substitutes are available. This way you keep the sweet but lose the calories. I will undoubtedly get letters and e-mails from "purists" who tell me that the sugar substitutes are just as bad as the sugar, and if I ever reach the point where I agree with them then I will revise this book and discuss 13 STOPs. But sprinkling some Splenda on top of fresh strawberries tastes just as good to me as drowning them in sugary syrup. The calories are limited to the almost negligible amount in the strawberries themselves. Ditto for some sweetener in coffee or tea, which I still enjoy but in modest and moderate measures. (Some sugar substitutes are supposed to cause memory loss and other health issues, but I can't remember what those are!)

2. **Refined or white flour and the products made from it.**
This pretty well eliminates most of the commercially prepared breads, buns, biscuits, and breaded products. This does not mean you should never and can never have bread, but if you must have it, get whole-grain bread made with flour that hasn't been so thoroughly processed that your digestive system thinks it hasn't eaten. Do keep in mind the big difference between pure "whole grain" and something that simply reports to be "wheat bread."

3. **Many fast foods.**
Notice I didn't say *all* fast foods, because the industry has acted in response to consumer demands and is beginning to make healthy options available on the menu. These days it isn't difficult at all to find healthy eating choices in fast-food restaurants, whether that be a salad, a low-carb wrap, or broiled or baked fish or chicken. I sparked quite some controversy in my state by remarking somewhat facetiously on a statewide radio call-in program that according to one doctor I knew, the motto was *If it comes through the car window, it isn't food!* Some folks in the fast-food

industry (particularly those with drive-through
windows) took offense and gave me an earful. I'd
made the remark half in jest, but there is a general
rule of thumb that if something is deep-fried in so
much fat it could leak through the sack, you'd be
better off ordering something else. If all else fails,
throw the food away, eat the sack, and at least
gain the fiber!

4. **Excess quantities of fatty meat.**
   Notice I didn't say that we shouldn't eat any meat
   or any fat. Doctors generally recognize that we
   need ample amounts of protein and even some fat
   in our diets. Despite having lost over a hundred
   pounds and gaining new strength and fitness, I still
   enjoy steak, pork ribs, all kinds of poultry, fish, and
   a variety of nuts, as well as fruits, vegetables, and
   grains.

   Don't let anyone tell you that a healthy diet is a
   boring diet—it most certainly is not! I perhaps enjoy
   the foods I eat now more than ever, because I've
   learned how to select them, savor them, and store
   them for energy rather than for fat.

5. **Starchy carbohydrates and vegetables such as
   potatoes and corn.**
   Since Arkansas is the number one rice producer in
   the nation, I'm not about to quit consuming rice (in
   part because I really love it, and in part because to
   do so would not be very smart politically!).
   Whenever possible, though, I eat whole-grain

brown unprocessed rice. I only occasionally eat potatoes or corn because both are high on the glycemic index scale, which means they tend to spike your blood sugar and increase cravings for additional food. This is even more of a problem for those of us fighting diabetes.

6. **Pasta.**

I like pasta and occasionally eat it, although I try to limit it to whole-grain pasta and avoid eating such food items early in the day when they can trigger increased appetite levels. But I have greatly limited starchy pastas for the reasons already noted.

7. **Trans-fatty acids and partially hydrogenated vegetable oil.**

Many food labels list "partially hydrogenated vegetable oil" as an ingredient. For the most part, you should treat these as if they read "poison—not for human consumption." Partially hydrogenated vegetable oil is essentially oleo margarine. It was engineered to help make food cheaper and longer lasting. At the time of its introduction, it was viewed as a very positive discovery—a replacement for butter with an extended shelf life. Problem was, while it did extend the shelf life of food, it cut short the lives of people who used it!

Out of necessity, I've dealt with some of the foods that we ought to stop depending on and eat less of. But what about the type of foods that we *should* eat? Some of this may depend on the particular food plan you're following, but here are some tips on what you should generally eat more of.

1. **Fruits and vegetables.**
   The rule of thumb is, *The more color, the fresher, and the leafier, the better.* Fortunately for me, I love fresh produce, and I've come to love fresh fruit–although this is a relatively newly acquired taste for me. A good guideline is that you should have at least five servings of fruits and vegetables a day; more is better. Lettuce, celery, broccoli, cauliflower, tomatoes, onions, cucumbers, asparagus, and green beans are just a few of the many delicious vegetables I enjoy. I used to hate asparagus (there was a time I would rather have eaten lawn clippings), but as my taste has changed I feel somewhat like the kid who has grown up and starts liking his broccoli. I wonder what was wrong with me all those years! (I still won't eat carrots, however. I'm not sure why. I just won't do it. I'm afraid if carrots were the only food my doctor prescribed, I'd have to get fat and die young.)

2. **Meats and seafood.**
   The good news for me is that I haven't had to quit eating meat, poultry, fish, or other forms of meat products, though I generally steer away from highly processed meat items. I have dramatically increased my appetite for and enjoyment of fresh fish, especially salmon. For reasons I don't fully comprehend, the foods I *do* eat taste better than

they ever have before, and even in much smaller quantities I derive more pleasure from having them than I did when I was eating an unlimited amount!

3. **Nuts and beans.**
When prepared properly, these can be a wonderful source of protein and fiber. They're quite healthy so long as they aren't prepared with enormous amounts of oil or consumed in large quantities.

4. **Dairy products and eggs.**
Modest amounts of cheese and low-fat or skim milk are excellent sources of calcium and protein. But you cannot have unlimited quantities of these, either. Eggs are also an excellent and delicious source of protein, but it's generally best to prepare them either poached or cooked with a noncalorie cooking spray as opposed to large amounts of butter. I often use olive oil for making scrambled eggs, or eat them hard-boiled.

This might be a good point to surprise you with my perspective on the government's role in what foods you should eat. I have stated on many occasions that I do not want the government to become the "grease police," dictating and ordering what people can and cannot eat. As much as I'm trying to watch my eating habits and adjust them to healthy choices, I do not believe that it's the government's role to tell me what I can or cannot eat. Nor is it the government's role to tell a private business owner who has put his own capital at risk to go into business what products he can or cannot legally serve just because someone might eat too much and get fat as a result.

Even worse is the flurry of ridiculous lawsuits in which people are lined up at the courthouse to sue fast-food restaurant chains for making their children fat! If parents are unaware that eating high-calorie fast food for breakfast, lunch, and dinner, every single day, can cause a caloric overload and a nutrition underload—well, those parents don't need to be in the courtroom as plaintiffs suing the fast-food vendor, they need to be in the courtroom as defendants for child abuse!

The McDonald's Corporation has been unfairly singled out for attack, the target of a documentary attempting to portray it as responsible for obesity by following a man who ate the unhealthiest choices on the menu three times a day for thirty days straight. The truth is, eating the unhealthiest options on *anyone's* menu three times a day for thirty days would make you sick!

McDonald's is no different from any other company—it's driven by consumer demand. That's why it launched its "go active" campaign in 2004, headed by renowned physiologist Bob Greene (Oprah Winfrey's personal trainer), and introduced a new line of healthy salads targeted at adults. Look at almost any fast-food menu today and you will find choices that are low-fat, low-carb, or sugar-free. Why? Because businesses exist to sell their products to consumers. They will sell what consumers buy! If you want to change the menu at McDonald's, don't change the law—change consumers' tastes and desires. By the summer of 2004, it was reported that McDonald's was selling more salads than french fries!

Suing fast-food chains for obesity is as absurd as suing the farmer who grew the wheat that became a bun, or the rancher who raised the cow that became a hamburger patty.

There is enough government intrusion into our lives without giving it a license to further invade our privacy, our liberties, and even our stupidity. No one is working harder right now than I am to try to change the health habits of a citizenry. But I continue to assert that the manner to best accomplish this is by positive leadership and incentives for proper behavior instead of penalties for improper behavior. I'm reminded of the admonition of Abraham Lincoln that "a government that can do everything for you is one that can take everything from you."

What if you're busy or it's hard to find good foods while traveling?

Remember our third STOP—STOP MAKING EXCUSES? Well, STOP making them! I travel a lot—almost every day. Many of my travels are day trips involving an early-morning departure with a return late that same night. Many other days I'm gone overnight, and I leave regularly for trips of several days each. Even though I can typically find things on menus that I can eat, I never assume it. I travel with a little soft-sided cooler everywhere I go. As the commercial for the American Express card says, "Don't leave home without it!" I don't. I even have several sizes, depending on the length of my trip and my likelihood of being able to stop or shop for healthy snacks or meals.

In my cooler, I carry bottled water, diet soft drinks, apples, strawberries, lean smoked chicken or turkey breast, cheese cubes, and similar items.

As a governor, I have people who are with me almost all the time, from staff to security. I could assign this task to others and claim it's beneath me to pack a little lunch box like a grade schooler, but I do it myself for several reasons. First, overeating is *my* problem, and *my* health is *my* responsibility. Packing my cooler is a reminder of my responsibility to make good choices today. Second, when I pack my cooler, I know exactly what's in it and how I've planned it to sustain me. I won't try to eat everything at once.

Do I get some strange looks carrying this around to hotels, in and out of cars and planes? Probably, but certainly fewer than when I was a hundred pounds overweight and getting eyed by people who feared they'd have to sit next to me on a crowded plane!

Once you get into the habit of packing your cooler, it will become second nature. It takes only a small bit of planning to keep your favorite items on hand at home. There are also meal-replacement options in shake or bar form—if all else fails. Packing and taking my cooler is now as much a part of my daily routine as brushing my teeth or buttoning my shirt.

Here's the deal: You can eat healthy if you want to, no matter where you are or who you are. I've done it while my wife and I took an eight-day cruise on the *Caribbean Princess* for our thirtieth wedding anniversary. (Now *that* was a challenge—there was abundant, fantastic food—but Princess lines, and no doubt others in the cruise business, work hard to have an incredible variety of appetizing, attractive, delicious, *and healthy* foods available at all times while also maintaining the most amazing onboard fitness center I've ever seen.) I've made it work from coast to coast and even while traveling overseas to Taiwan, Japan, and Europe.

No matter where you are, it is crucial to make the best food choices for your body, and that means you absolutely must

STOP FUELING WITH CONTAMINATED FOOD.

DEAR GOVERNOR HUCKABEE,

I'm a young Spanish boy that has read about your spectacular loss of weight in the Spanish newspapers. I believe that you are very brave because I am young, but I have lost 43 kilos. You must have a lot of will force to make this and it's a very important thing in a governor. You are an example for your state and for the world. Thank you and greetings from Spain.

Madrid, Spain

STOP 11

STOP Allowing Food to Be a Reward

If I could accumulate all the weight I've lost over a lifetime of yo-yo dieting, I could probably turn it into an anchor and hold the *Queen Mary 2* in place during heavy swells! Losing weight and then regaining it generally results in not only gaining back the weight you've lost, but adding even more as well. If you're reading this book, the pattern is already familiar to you, and you likely have experienced the same level of frustration. There is also a strong likelihood that this makes you skeptical of ever making fitness and health a permanent, lifelong experience.

Even now, you fear you will once again be a "starter" but not a "finisher." As you review some of these important STOPs that you must make in order to enact true lifestyle change, the next one seems obvious enough. Still, I must confess I never adhered to it until I was ready to pursue a life of fitness rather than a life of dieting.

From the time we are tots, most of us have celebrated special occasions and special events with a reward of foods that are rarely nutritious or healthy. The most obvious example is the traditional birthday cake, usually accompanied by large scoops of ice cream. Birthdays were special occasions in my household, but not because my family went all-out to observe them. In fact, they were a somewhat low-key affair from the standpoint of elaborate "bells and whistles" and expensive gifts. But one thing always marked my birthday in the Huckabee household: a small chocolate cake from Joe's City Bakery in Hope, Arkansas (which, by the way, was the *only* bakery in Hope, Arkansas, in the 1950s and 1960s!).

My mother was an excellent cook gloriously gifted with taking the staples of "Southern haute cuisine" and turning them into excellent pies and cakes. But for a poor kid, anything store-bought just seemed extra special and marked sacrifice on the part of the family.

I can close my eyes right now and still remember the distinctive aroma, texture, and taste of the little chocolate cake that I would get on my birthday from Joe's City Bakery. It was easy to begin associating the pleasant nature of a birthday with the anticipation of that special treat.

Most rewards and celebrations of milestones in my family were indeed food-related. If I went to the doctor and didn't scream, cry, or kick the nurse in the shin, I was rewarded with a nice lollipop and might even be allowed to get a Cherry Coke at the soda fountain at Cox's Drug Store on Second Street. When accompanying my mother to the grocery store, my reward for succeeding in navigating the store aisles without knocking over major displays of canned goods might be selecting a candy bar at the checkout stand. Victories on the Little League baseball field were marked with a snow cone or, in the case of a major victory, maybe even an ice cream cone at the local Dairy Queen. Even describing it forty years later evokes pleasant and special memories.

By the same token, penalties for improper behavior often included having desserts or various treats withheld. I was never sent to bed without my supper during those formative years, but sometimes I had to forgo desserts or treats if I had misbehaved. I much preferred the old-fashioned spanking (which I received regularly) for various infractions. I've often said I was raised in a very patriotic family by an exceptionally patriotic father who "laid on the stripes so that I could see the stars!"

Childhood rewards of food for successful behavior didn't change but only transitioned during adolescence and even during my adult years. From the simple rewards of a cookie or a piece of candy during childhood, later "pizza parties" or hamburger cookouts became part of marking special events or happy occasions in adolescence. As an adult, it would be a steak dinner in a nice restaurant, with an appetizer, dessert, and the works!

I'm not saying we should never mark our special occasions with treats. But we may have conditioned ourselves to associate pleasant moments with indulging ourselves in every imaginable food—most of which are the unhealthiest choices we can make. It is as if we believe that great moments, great accomplishments, special occasions, and significant milestones in life are tied to an orgy of eating unlimited quantities of the things we are normally told to limit.

Having spent a lifetime associating unhealthy food with good behavior, is it any wonder that changing our lifestyle is a significant challenge?

As I contemplated one day why I had failed on so many previous diet attempts, it suddenly hit me like a cream pie in the face! I sat alone and actually started laughing out loud.

During my previous attempts to lose weight, I deprived myself of certain foods, and throughout the process I genuinely felt I was *being deprived*. With an almost masochistic sense of sacrifice, I dutifully consumed the low-fat vegetables while avoiding all the things I normally associated with happiness and success. I felt I was painfully punishing myself as I lost pounds and inches. As I inched toward my target weight, however, I anticipated arriving at my destination and celebrating the victory. And I had been conditioned since I was in diapers that there can be *no* celebration without a vast array of my favorite foods.

As crazy as it sounds, I often celebrated reaching my target weight by convincing myself that it would be perfectly appropriate to mark the weight loss with a "special dinner" in which I ate all the things I hadn't touched in months! I sat down and enjoyed the delicious pleasures I associated with success. The combination of a happy occasion with an almost orgasmic surrender to all the various tastes associated with happy occasions affirmed that eating—especially eating junk food—was "happiness," and eating those things which I considered "healthy" was "punishment"!

Who of us in our right minds wants to spend a lifetime feeling punished?

My wife and I have a home on Lake Greeson in southwest Arkansas, a beautiful body of water in the foothills of the Ouachita Mountains. When I'm there, I often take early-morning walks or runs through the woods. In the spring and summer, my senses are awakened with the captivating aroma of fresh honeysuckle. One day as I walked and devoured that familiar fragrance, it occurred to me why that sweet smell brought such a feeling of peace and well-being.

As a small child, I loved summer mornings. I'd eat cereal, watch *Captain Kangaroo*, and then head outside while the dew was still on the ground to cool my always bare feet. I'd join up with the other kids in the neighborhood to collect the soda pop bottles in the streets and ditches in a little red wagon. We'd then turn them in at the Piggly Wiggly supermarket for the deposit money. Twice a week we'd have enough so that when George Walden, the milkman, came through the neighborhood delivering milk, we'd be able to buy orange drink and chocolate milk right off the truck. We'd spend the rest of the day outside, playing baseball, riding bikes, or playing with a garden hose to get cool in the afternoon heat. But each morning began with the same sweet honeysuckle aroma. As I walked now through the woods and caught the whiff of honeysuckle, the wonderful memories and powerful emotions of a simpler time overwhelmed me. The smell of the honeysuckle brought back to me the peaceful and worry-free existence of a six-year-old kid in Hope, Arkansas, releasing me from a thousand pressures of being governor—I wasn't worried about a thing! I was conditioned to associate the aroma of honeysuckle with something pleasant!

This single revelation has made a significant difference in my ability to adjust to a new lifestyle. My previous failures were in large part the result of a lifetime of *conditioning myself for failure* and not having any idea how to be *conditioned for success and fitness*!

Most of our plans to lose weight focus on the *steps* we need to take to successfully lose weight. Unfortunately, few of them focus on the STOPs we must make to change the very conditioning that has caused us a lifetime of chronic failure. Chronic failure and the inability to achieve health and fitness become permanent punishment.

For those people who grew up being rewarded with carrots and celery instead of cake, maybe none of this registers. But quite frankly, if you grew up being rewarded with carrots and celery, you probably didn't buy this book anyway! You are reading someone else's copy wondering *What's the big deal?* because you have never struggled with weight like some of us and can't relate to these challenges.

This particular STOP will require some imagination and, frankly, some hard work on your part. I'm not necessarily suggesting that you announce to your small children that they will no longer receive a birthday cake and instead will be given a plate of broccoli with a candle positioned on it for their next significant moment! Chances are they would report you as an abuser if you attempted to make such a radical change so quickly. But do begin shifting away from this "tradition of condition" that ties achievement to indulgence.

Be creative! If a friend of yours needs special attention, consider taking him to a movie instead of out for a double fudge sundae. Or give her a gift certificate for a CD or DVD instead of one for pizza or ice cream.

As you begin to reward yourself and even contemplate a new level of fitness, anticipate that *your* reward will be clothes that fit and a day at the ocean, where you may not be mistaken for a beached whale. Plan a trip where you will fly in coach and actually be able to get in and out of the seat without twisting. You won't require a seat belt extension, and you won't find yourself sitting with your arms folded across your chest the entire trip because resting them at your sides means putting them in your neighbor's face.

To be fair, you have spent a lifetime being conditioned to celebrate with eating. You need to begin *reconditioning* yourself to break these bad habits. But it should be easier now that you are aware of *why* you've found it so difficult to overcome the extraordinary urge to gorge yourself on fattening foods. Hopefully you will be able to do something about it and

STOP ALLOWING FOOD TO BE A REWARD.

DEAR GOVERNOR,

I just had to write you to offer my heartfelt congratulations on your recent "transformation." I read your wonderful story and I must say I was most impressed by what you have accomplished, particularly since you did it the old-fashioned way–with faith, prayer, and willpower. You look great, and I'm sure you feel that way, too. Although I'm not a fellow Arkansan, I'm proud of you.

Mississippi

STOP 12

STOP Neglecting Your Spiritual Health

A common characteristic of every 12-step program with which I'm familiar is the affirmation that without assistance from and adherence to a higher power, we are destined to fail.

Of my many motivations to move toward a concept of forever fit, the primary one was in fact *faith*.

Before you get spooked and close the book fearing you are about to get a preachy sermon, relax! At the end of the book, I will share with you more about my convictions regarding faith. But for now, I simply want you to recognize the importance of your *spiritual* health as well as your *physical* health.

Chances are, your primary purpose in seeking a new level of health and fitness is the way you look, the way you feel, or maybe simply to achieve a level of well-being. You want to live longer and be happier. Nothing is wrong with this, but you need to begin seeing yourself in the larger context (no pun intended). Before you try to fit into your world (and your clothes), think about fitting into a larger scheme of life. It's my hope that you will appreciate the need for taking care of yourself for reasons larger than those gleaned from your last medical checkup.

Assume for a moment there is no God, higher power, universal force, or anything metaphysical that exists outside the realm of the five senses—touch, taste, hearing, smell, and sight. If that is in fact the case, and life is a mere biological accident, then you might as well "eat, drink, and be merry, for tomorrow you die." Such things as personal achievement or a sense of legacy are just games if we are nothing more than independent configurations of human cells.

But let's assume we're more than that. Regardless of your own personal convictions as to the nature of the supernatural and the spiritual, let's assume that the incredible creation around us does in fact have a Creator and that the design we see in all living things does in fact have a Designer. If there is a purpose for the manner in which our bodies have been designed, then there is probably a plan for how those bodies are to be serviced and cared for. This assumption doesn't require a great leap of faith on anyone's part. You don't have to pray three hours a day or chant loudly enough to wake the neighbors to understand what I'm talking about.

Every time I buy an appliance or electronic gadget, it comes with a detailed book of instructions. The first several pages are usually warnings of the obvious, such as: "Do not use the electric toaster in the bathtub" (something I would never have thought of had they not warned me!). It usually proceeds to sections outlining the proper use of the item based on the manner in which it was created. (I am one of those geeks who actually reads the manual before operating the equipment. Which means I typically know much less about how it actually works than my wife, who pulls it out of the box, hooks it up the way she thinks it should work, and then refers to the manual only if something doesn't function the way she expected.)

Nevertheless, not only does the design have a designer, but there are specific instructions on how to use the device for optimum performance. It should not come as a big surprise that the amazing capacity of our human bodies is best served when we realize that it has instructions on how it can best be utilized for peak performance.

Before I could make any permanent changes in my own lifestyle, I had to accept the fact that I was not being a good steward (manager, caretaker) of the body God had given me. While I could make many cute jokes as to why this was the case, it did not diminish the fact I would likely meet my Maker sooner than I intended—not because of *His* design, but because of my dereliction of duty in taking care of what He had created.

Properly cared for, the human body is an amazing machine! No camera has ever been created that has the full range of optical capacity the human eye enjoys. No electronic device can yet surpass or even mimic the amazing capacity of the human ear to hear and distinguish a range of frequencies. While certain animals may have a more distinctive capacity for smell, no electronic or human-made device has ever equaled the version found in the nose. While robots are able to mimic many human functions, the most delicate surgical procedures still require some level of touch from the physician for accuracy and effectiveness. The ability to taste is a marvel into itself. (In fact, our incredible ability to taste and enjoy what we taste is one of the reasons you're reading this book right now!) If you were nothing more than a machine, you would be able to exist on a bland fuel that offered no sense of pleasure or aesthetic enjoyment and which could be purchased like gasoline at the pump. You would consume only what was needed for your capacity and energy demands.

The human heart and circulation together represent one of the most sophisticated pumping systems ever imagined. Our digestive system is without question amazing and combines the capacities to extract energy from fuel and to efficiently dispose of any waste. Our brain and central nervous system represent a level of advanced circuitry that eclipses any computer devised in terms of its complex scope and magnitude, as well as its capacity for multitasking.

Now, if you still want to believe you are all on your own, have no spiritual life, and are nothing more than physical configuration of DNA or animated protoplasm, then so be it. But success in the 12 STOPs includes recognizing that you must *STOP neglecting your spiritual health* and include it as a vital part of your quest to be the best.

The key to succeeding at this last STOP is simply recognizing you are not alone in your goal, don't have to be, and, for success, probably can't be.

A key element of success in changing bad habits is accountability to others. If you and a friend challenge each other to eat healthy food then go out to eat, you wouldn't dare order a "death by chocolate" dessert—doing so would break your agreement *and* your credibility. All alone back at home, however, you might remember where you stashed that package of Oreos. You might indulge yourself in a "package of passionate pleasure" because "no one is looking."

When you stop neglecting your spiritual health, you will realize that someone is *always* watching, and you will begin to understand that your accountability is not only to yourself, your doctor, your family, and the friends with whom you have committed to better health, but also to your Creator and your God, to the one who is present when all others are gone, who is awake when all others are asleep, and who is always watching even when others are looking the other way. Don't take this as a negative "Big Brother is watching" and "He's going to bust my chops if I fall." View this important part of your life as having a *friend* who will never leave your side and who is willing to stay up with you all day and all night to help you be a *winner*. Furthermore, this friend is not trying to condemn you or heap guilt on you but rather is interested in your well-being for *your* sake. He wants you to receive all of the benefits and pleasures that are possible through the instrument of your body, which He created and provided for you.

Some people want to lose weight because they hate themselves and hope that by changing they will develop a better self-image. This book is about getting healthy—and doing it not because you see yourself as worthless, but because you believe you're worth improving! Truth is, if you really hate yourself when you're fat, you'll probably hate yourself even if you're thin. It's not your weight that's giving you the bad self-image; it's the self-image that is giving you the weight!

Your Creator wants you to derive all the benefit and pleasures of the body He made for you, and since it's *His* design, He does know how to coach you for optimum performance. I hope you will burn this last STOP clearly into your mind:

STOP NEGLECTING YOUR SPIRITUAL HEALTH.

DEAR GOVERNOR,

It was great to see your story about your personal, physical transformation on a syndicated television show up here in Michigan.

Michigan

APPENDIX I

Tips for the First Twelve Days

The first days of any change in your life are the most challenging. John Bingham, who has written several books on running and calls himself "The Penguin" because of his running/walking style, has a motto that I embrace and identify with: *The miracle isn't that I finished; the miracle is that I had the courage to start.*

You've decided to *do something*. You're a little nervous, because you've probably tried and failed before—maybe many times. Remember, this time you're going to succeed because you're not going to quit. This is not a program or a "plan." It's committing to simply taking care of yourself, and you start today, but understand it will take the rest of your life to succeed.

Here are some simple yet practical tips for the first twelve days. On each of these twelve days, begin by rereading a chapter and reflecting on these questions:

1. How does this STOP relate to *my* experience?

2. What is the major lesson I learn from this STOP?
3. On a scale of 1 through 10, how hard is this STOP going to be for me?
4. What specifically would I STOP today to live out this principle?

You will make it!

DAY ONE: STOP PROCRASTINATING

* Reread chapter 1.
* Get up fifteen minutes earlier.
* Engage in twelve minutes of physical activity (not too difficult or strenuous!). Remember, the issue is *time*, not intensity. A slow walk or light bike riding is fine.
* Tell a friend what you're doing.
* Drink lots of water throughout the day.
* Having chosen a food/calorie plan, stick faithfully to it, no matter what!
* Here are a few food guidelines to help you:
    * No sugar!
    * Unless you're having medically supervised meal replacements, eat a protein breakfast (eggs, perhaps), a salad or steamed vegetables for lunch, and, for dinner, broiled, baked, or grilled chicken or fish with steamed or raw vegetables.
    * If you have to have a snack, have an apple or some berries.
* Stay busy with plenty of activity.

DAY TWO: STOP MAKING EXCUSES

* Reread chapter 2.
* Repeat everything from Day One.

* Stick faithfully to your planned food intake—*no* cheating!
* Make a list of the reasons you've told yourself you'll fail—then laugh at the list and promise not to obey your past patterns.

DAY THREE: STOP SITTING ON THE COUCH
* Reread chapter 3.
* Repeat the basics from Day One.
* Make a list of the kinds of activity you would likely enjoy.
* Don't sit in your normal chair in the family room.
* Don't allow yourself to watch television other than the news, and again, not from your favorite chair! (It's about breaking patterns or habits.)

DAY FOUR: STOP IGNORING SIGNALS FROM YOUR BODY
* Reread chapter 4.
* Repeat the basics.
* Review your medical records and doctor's advice.
* Add up your health care costs from the previous year. Ask yourself how much savings you would have seen in doctor, hospital, and medical expenses if you had been healthy. Make a list of what you would use that much money for.

DAY FIVE: STOP LISTENING TO DESTRUCTIVE CRITICISM
* Reread chapter 5.
* Repeat the basics.
* Call an old friend you haven't talked to in a while and share what you're doing and why.
* Make a list of ten benefits you'll get from being healthy.

DAY 6: STOP EXPECTING IMMEDIATE SUCCESS

* Reread chapter 6.
* Repeat the basics.
* Write down three major health goals you want to achieve *one year* from now.

DAY SEVEN: STOP WHINING

* Reread chapter 7.
* Repeat the basics.
* Make a list of friends and co-workers who are negative—then promise yourself to avoid them and not listen to them.
* List five things you are truly grateful for.

DAY EIGHT: STOP MAKING EXCEPTIONS

* Reread chapter 8.
* Repeat the basics.
* List the upcoming special events and holidays and make plans for *not* overeating—alternative foods, not going to the event, what have you.
* Think of at least two occasions *today* when you have said no to a temptation, and reflect on how it made you feel to overcome the desire.

DAY NINE: STOP STORING PROVISIONS FOR FAILURE

* Reread chapter 9.
* Repeat the basics.
* Spend twenty minutes looking for and getting rid of unhealthy foods that you shouldn't be eating, including any hidden stashes in your desk drawers, car, and cabinets.

* Tell family members where you were hiding "failure food," and tell them you need their help in staying away from it.

DAY TEN: STOP FUELING WITH CONTAMINATED FOOD
* Reread chapter 10.
* Repeat the basics.
* Spend twenty minutes reading the labels of foods in your house and seeing how many of those things contain the "bad boys"– sugar, high-fructose corn syrup, or partially hydrogenated vegetable oil.
* List eight to ten healthy foods you like or at least can tolerate, and be sure to always have two or three on hand.

DAY ELEVEN: STOP ALLOWING FOOD TO BE A REWARD
* Reread chapter 11.
* Repeat the basics.
* Make a list of events, holidays, and special occasions coming up in the next three months and write down alternatives to the preferred food choices for such occasions.
* Write down three of your most vivid memories of great moments in your childhood and note if food was a part of them.

DAY TWELVE: STOP NEGLECTING YOUR SPIRITUAL HEALTH
* Reread chapter 12.
* Repeat the basics.
* Spend at least ten minutes reading a favorite inspirational book– the Bible, a devotional book, poetry, or another special volume.

* Write one or two paragraphs about why you need to be a better caretaker of your body.
* Make an appointment to talk with your minister, priest, rabbi, or trusted friend to ask for prayers and encouragement as you seek to change your health.

Dear Governor,

I have struggled with weight loss for several years, but have not lost all hope yet. Your comments were very encouraging. I thought that not only were you an inspiration to many Americans facing weight loss issues, but you made some very important statements concerning leadership philosophy that are missing in many politicians today. I'm a seventh-grade teacher, math department head at my school, a military spouse, and a mom. I admire people who take a stand for the good of children.

New York

APPENDIX II

What Government Should and Shouldn't Do

The health care system in America is the best in the world, but unfortunately it rests on a faulty and ultimately fatal foundation. Our system is built on the premise of spending money to *treat* disease—yet many diseases are in fact absolutely *preventable*. This premise governs not only public health plans such as Medicaid and Medicare but also private insurance plans. Companies try to provide employees with comprehensive health benefits, but find it increasingly difficult to do so because of spiraling costs that grow in gross disproportion to the rate of inflation and other expenses. Governors in all fifty states, be they Democrat or Republican, universally agree that the Medicaid program operated by states (the program originally designed to take care of our poor and needy citizens) has reached an unsustainable level of costs; without significant reform, it will bankrupt state budgets in the very near future. During my first eight years as governor of

Arkansas, our own Medicaid budget has grown from six hundred million dollars a year to over three billion.

Most medical professionals are trained to treat illness and disease, but often they do not train patients and clients in healthy behavior.

Most insurance plans will cover the hundreds of thousands of dollars for open-heart surgery or for the costly treatment of and rehabilitation from a stroke, but will not contribute one dime for weight loss programs or fitness regimens that might have prevented the heart attack or stroke in the first place.

I have embarked on a mission to challenge the faulty thinking of our current system that could result in a complete change in the paradigm of health care in America.

In spring 2004, Arkansas launched the Healthy Arkansas Initiative.

The concept is simple—we want to create a culture of health by encouraging healthy behavior and choices, and devise a whole menu of incentives for people who make those choices. Dr. Fay Boozman, director of the Arkansas Department of Health, put it best: "We need to stop treating snakebites and start killing snakes."

In the first phase of Healthy Arkansas, we have targeted the three specific areas of behavior that can produce the most dramatic results. Studies show that those who maintain a normal body weight, get regular exercise (at least thirty minutes per day, three times a week), and abstain from the use of tobacco will likely add an additional thirteen years to their life spans. Moreover, not only will the *quantity* of your life be extended, but its *quality* will be dramatically enhanced by those three simple behaviors as well.

Beginning in 2005, state employees in Arkansas who are willing to undergo a health risk assessment to help gauge the incidence of risky behaviors will be given a discount of up to twenty dollars per month from their state employee health insurance. In addition, we are looking for other means to provide incentives for people to take charge of their own health—which not only proves beneficial to the individual but will be a tremendous cost savings to the employer.

Ultimately, it is my hope and goal that Healthy Arkansas will spread like a highly contagious but benevolent virus that could become the genesis of "Healthy America." I'd like to see all fifty states find creative ways to reward positive behavior rather than continually pay absurd amounts of money for the catastrophic results of bad behavior and health.

Many people rightly argue that we do not need the government monitoring or controlling what happens in the privacy of our own homes. Interestingly, some of the same people who demand that government stay out of our bedrooms are demanding that it take over the kitchen! They are suggesting that we create a whole system of penalties and prohibitions on unhealthy eating that range from an extra tax on fatty foods to an outright ban of certain types of foods.

Historically, telling liberty-loving Americans what they can and cannot do has not proven very successful. What *does* work is changing the culture so that individual choices become cultural choices and ultimately the behavioral norm. Smoking is increasingly considered boorish and invasive behavior, not so much because of a government-sponsored ban as because people are more aware of the health risk and find the practice annoying and disgusting. Consumers have insisted on nonsmoking hotel rooms, restaurants, airlines, and public buildings.

Personally, I hope the tobacco habit dies a quick and ugly

death, and the sooner, the better! But in those instances in which government has attempted to unilaterally restrict personal choices in private business or private homes, the battle has been shifted from a discussion of health to one of personal rights.

In my own state, we are seeking to find positive ways to encourage our employees to make healthy decisions. To promote exercise, we gave every employee in the governor's office who wanted one a personal pedometer. This is a simple device you hook on to your belt to measure the number of steps you take in a day. A goal of ten thousand steps per day (the equivalent of about five miles) is a good benchmark for the kind of daily exercise that will help you develop personal fitness and lose weight. We created a contest in which the employee who walked the most steps was able to use the much-coveted parking place of our chief of staff for a two-week period.

It occurred to me that we were forced to allow our smoking employees to have at least two fifteen-minute breaks per day so that they might indulge in their unhealthy and deadly habit. Perhaps we should encourage healthy behavior by giving time to those employees who wish to take a walking or exercise break. Even though our offices are completely smoke-free and have been since the day I took the oath of office, smoking staff members were being accommodated (albeit outside the doors of the State Capitol). Now we have several employees in "walking groups" who on a daily basis take brisk walks in or around the Capitol. We've discovered that healthier employees are more alert, more productive, make fewer mistakes, and have fewer days of absenteeism.

As I have stated on numerous occasions, we do not need the government to become the "grease police," dictating what size cheeseburger the law will allow or taxing obese people at a different rate than thin people because of the likelihood of additional health care costs associated with obesity.

My own personal journey of discovering the joy of health through sensible eating and exercise has heightened my sense of mission as both a public official and a private citizen to help other individuals and to lead in discovering *creative and positive* public policies that will hopefully result in the ultimate goal of Healthy Arkansas, with a changed culture of health.

DEAR GOVERNOR,

Your story is certainly inspiring, and I pray that you remain healthy also. Congratulations on your accomplishment.

Georgia

In addition to the perspective of stewardship, my faith gave me the basis for insisting that accountability be a part of my lifestyle plan. This accountability is not only to other human beings such as my doctor, nutritionist, and family, but also to the God whom I believe is with me without fail at all times. A sense of His perpetual presence was tremendous encouragement and provided genuine strength when I needed it most.

Through each stage of success, my faith enabled me to experience satisfaction knowing that not only was I improving my behavior but I was actually bringing pleasure to my Creator, God, Father.

I would never seek to impose my deep personal convictions on others and sincerely hope that a discussion of the spiritual does not come across as judgmental, arrogant, or self-serving. I simply believe it disingenuous to discuss my journey (and my hope for *yours*) without telling "the truth, the *whole* truth, and nothing but the truth."

APPENDIX III

The Faith Factor

While I'm convinced that the essentials of this book can be applied whether you work from a spiritual perspective or not, attention to spiritual health is a vital part of my own experience and may in fact be necessary for most people in achieving lifetime of success. It was my goal (and that of the publisher) avoid being "preachy" and not create what some would disas a "religious" book. I would be less than honest, however did not give some credit to the role of faith in my own quehealth. If you are offended by such discussion, you are cefree to pass up reading this portion of the book. But this other personal choices, is your decision to make.

A major part of my motivation in wanting to be he sense of stewardship to God as well as to my family. believe that I'm not a biological accident but rather t a creative process of an omniscient God, I came escapable conclusion that my personal lifestyle ch direct contradiction to the very way I had been cr